Examinations of Competency to Stand Trial

Foundations in Mental Health Case Law

Richard I. Frederick
Richart L. DeMier
Karin Towers

Professional Resource Press
Sarasota, Florida

Published by
Professional Resource Press
(An Imprint of the Professional Resource Exchange, Inc.)
Post Office Box 15560
Sarasota, FL 34277-1560

Printed in the United States of America

The copy editor for this book was Patricia Rockwood, the managing editor was Debbie Fink, the production coordinator was Laurie Girsch, the text designer was Deirdre DeLay, and the cover designer was Jami Stinnet.

Library of Congress Cataloging-in-Publication Data

Frederick, Richard I., date.
　Examinations of competency to stand trial: foundations in mental health case law / Richard I. Frederick, Richart L. DeMier, Karin Towers.
　　p. cm.
　Includes bibliographical references.
　ISBN 1-56887-084-1 (alk. paper)
　1. Competency to stand trial--United States. 2. Forensic psychiatry--United States. 3. Psychology, Forensic--United States. I. DeMier, Richart L., date. II. Towers, Karin, date. III. Title.
KF9242.F74 2004
342.73 04--dc22

2003058422

Table of Contents

Section 3 *(Continued)*

Section 4 - Incompetent Defendants 137

Section 5 - Amnesia & Competency 219

Appendices 255

Introduction to the Volume

In assessing competency to stand trial, mental health professionals must marry clinical judgments with the legal standards that define competency. In order to develop conclusions that are useful and understandable to the courts, clinicians must discern and address those core issues of competency articulated by courts. In essence, judicial guidelines concerning the nature and scope of competency to stand trial determine how the evaluation proceeds.

A number of excellent books have addressed the process of completing clinical assessments of the competency of criminal defendants. In doing so, the authors of these books generally provide the legal definitions of competency and incompetency, and then delineate clinical methods of evaluating relevant deficits and abilities by standard and specialized methods of psychological or psychiatric assessment. This book differs in that its *primary* focus is how courts construe competency and not how clinicians should conduct examinations. By exploring the thinking of courts in resolving procedural and substantive issues related to competency, we believe the ultimate effect will be that clinicians can better identify those areas meriting special attention when assessing competency.

As an example, a U.S. Supreme Court case that clearly defines mental competency to stand trial is *Dusky v. United States* (1960).[1] In *Dusky*, the Supreme Court held that a defendant was competent if he "has sufficient present ability to consult with his lawyer with a reasonable degree of rational understanding - and whether he has a rational as well as factual understanding of the proceedings against him." Dusky received a clinical examination

---

[1] *Dusky v. United States* (1960) refers to the decision by the United States Supreme Court. Dusky appealed a U.S. Court of Appeals decision about what constituted competency. The Supreme Court granted a hearing on the matter in 1959 and rendered a decision in 1960.

of competency prior to standing trial on charges of kidnapping and rape. On appeal, the Supreme Court concluded there was something fundamentally flawed in the process of determining competency to stand trial. In essence, the Supreme Court held that even though the clinician had completed a statutorily defined examination, he had nonetheless failed to capture the most essential elements of what courts must consider in making decisions about competency. The key characteristics of Dusky's clinical examination highlighted a shortcoming in the law. Prior to *Dusky*, clinicians had no effective means to anticipate this issue; after *Dusky*, any clinician who did not incorporate the Supreme Court's directive would fail to serve the court that ordered the examination. Given this potential problem, the goal of this book is to review important judicial decisions that should guide the thinking of clinicians who evaluate and report on criminal competencies.

In decisions like *Dusky*, the Supreme Court and all lower appellate courts generally render opinions based on an analysis of the facts at hand and by incorporating legal foundations from previous appellate decisions (i.e., finding precedents in case law). In determining whether to address an issue on appeal, courts generally determine whether the issue is one of settled law (previously heard and decided) or whether a new application of law is required to address an inequity. In addition to *Dusky*, the Supreme Court and other appellate courts have addressed many finer points of what constitutes competency and have spoken to many aspects of how competency should be addressed.

In this book, we will review case law pertaining to many facets of competency to stand trial. We have sorted these cases into five sections. The first section - Standards of Competency - examines basic legal principles of competency to stand trial. The second section - Thresholds of Competency Examinations - concerns important secondary principles of the adjudication of competency (e.g., those instances in which a competency examination must be ordered). The next section - Constitutional and Judicial Considerations - reviews cases that reflect points on which mental health professionals and legal decision makers commonly diverge; these cases inform the clinician about the court's perspective. The fourth section - Incompetent Defendants - involves cases concerning what should happen with defendants who are found incompetent to stand trial. The final section - Amnesia and Competency - examines cases that reflect a variety of perspectives on defendants who claim amnesia for the crimes for which they are charged.

For each case, we present a *brief*, which is a concise summary of the case. A brief encapsulates the essential facts of the case, the issue before the court, the court's analysis, and the holding. Following the brief, we present Edited Excerpts of discussion by the court, as an amplification of the reasons it reached its holding. After each section, we provide Implications for Examiners, remarking upon how the courts' rulings should be applied within clinical examinations.

This book specifically concerns competency to stand trial. Although issues concerning competency to confess and competency to be sentenced are related to competency to stand trial, they fall outside the scope of this book. Interested readers may wish to consult *Miranda v. Arizona* and *Colorado v. Connelly* (cases concerning competency to confess) and *Saddler v. United States* and *Ford v. Wainwright* (cases concerning competency to be sentenced). Full citations for these cases are in Appendix A (pp. 257-260).

Edited Excerpts

Edited Excerpts are intended to distill the essence of judicial reasoning regarding the elements of competency to stand trial. Many cases are appealed on more than one issue. We have omitted the text of the case that is not directly relevant to the issue of competency to stand trial. Additionally, legal decisions often contain content and format that make them difficult to read. In our Edited Excerpts, we have liberally excised text and altered format to improve readability. These changes are generally not evident. As an example, consider the following passage from *Godinez v. Moran*:

> A criminal defendant may not be tried unless he is competent, Pate v. Robinson, 383 U.S. 375, 378 (1966), and he may not waive his right to counsel or plead guilty unless he does so "competently and intelligently," Johnson v. Zerbst, 304 U.S. 458, 468 (1938); accord, Brady v. United States, 397 U.S. 742, 758 (1970). In Dusky v. United States, 362 U.S. 402 (1960) (per curiam), we held that the standard for competence to stand trial is whether the defendant has "sufficient present ability to consult with his lawyer with a reasonable degree of rational understanding" and has "a rational as well as factual understanding of the proceedings against him." Ibid. (internal quotation marks omitted).

What we present in this book reads as follows:

A criminal defendant may not be tried unless he is competent (*Pate*), and he may not waive his right to counsel or plead guilty unless he does so "competently and intelligently" *(Johnson v. Zerbst)*. In *Dusky*, we held that the standard for competence to stand trial is whether the defendant has "sufficient present ability to consult with his lawyer with a reasonable degree of rational understanding" and has "a rational as well as factual understanding of the proceedings against him."

To present the court's decision in a more readable fashion, we also eliminate the court's notations of changed text (e.g., brackets or ellipses). For example, a sentence which, in the original text, might read "The defendant is reported to have said: '[W]e saw that [they] . . . were alone' " would read in this book: "The defendant is reported to have said: 'We saw that they were alone.' "

Sometimes we will change the text or insert words to improve readability. For example, consider the following text from *Jackson v. Indiana*:

> "We therefore must turn to the question whether, because of the pendency of the criminal charges that triggered the State's invocation of 9-1706a, Jackson was deprived of substantial rights to which he would have been entitled under either of the other two state commitment statutes."

Additions and changes to the text to improve readability are noted by brackets:

> "We therefore must turn to the question whether, because of the pendency of the criminal charges that triggered the State's invocation of [statute], Jackson was deprived of substantial rights to which he would have been entitled under either of [Indiana's] other two state commitment statutes."

Consequently, it is extremely important that the reader understand that our Edited Excerpts cannot be cited to accurately reflect what is in the original text of the decision. Readers who wish to cite the original text of a case must obtain the published case. Within our treatment of each case, we have provided the proper citation to obtain the original text. A list of full case citations is provided in Appendix A (pp. 257-260).

Jurisdictional Scope

In the United States, there are two types of controlling law - statutory law and case law. Statutory law comprises laws enacted by state or federal legislatures. For example, federal criminal law is codified in the U.S. Code, Section 18. Other types of law (e.g., real estate law and bankruptcy law) are also written into statute and enacted by legislatures. Statutory law also includes rules of evidence and defines procedures to be followed by the judiciary in the resolution of disputes.

Case law refers to the body of law promulgated by state and federal judicial systems. When the meaning or appropriate application of law is in dispute, individuals or groups appeal to higher courts for resolution. The party who raises an issue is generally known as the petitioner or appellant, and the party who counters is the respondent or appellee.

The cases in this book originated at a state or federal trial court. Most involved issues appealed to higher courts. States and the federal government have sets of successively higher appellate courts which culminate in the highest court in the state or, in the federal system, the United States Supreme Court. The names of appellate courts vary among jurisdictions. For example, most state systems culminate in a state Supreme Court, but New York's highest court is the Court of Appeals; lower New York courts are called Supreme Courts.

In the federal government, trial courts are called district courts. Decisions of a district court can be appealed to one of the 11 Circuit Courts of Appeals. Decisions of circuit courts can be appealed to the United States Supreme Court.

Most cases begin at the trial court level. As the result of appeals, the case may be heard by courts of successively higher authority. When there is an allegation that a state law conflicts with federal law, or when a party contends that a right bestowed by the United States Constitution has been violated, state cases can be appealed within the federal judiciary.

The resulting body of case law provides guidance regarding the interpretation and application of law. Decisions from case law may have either jurisdictional authority or persuasive authority. Jurisdictional authority means the holding of the appellate court becomes law in the jurisdiction controlled by that court. For example, *United States v. Greer* is a federal appellate decision issued by the Court of Appeals for the Fifth Circuit. Unless subsequently overturned by the United States Supreme Court, the ruling is controlling law in the Fifth Circuit.

In some cases, a court is presented with an issue or question that has not previously arisen in that jurisdiction. In such cases, a court might look to the opinion of another court for analysis or guidance. Arguments and decisions from another jurisdiction may establish persuasive authority for a particular position, but they are not binding. It is for this reason we include *Wieter v. Settle*, a District Court decision that has often been cited by trial and appellate courts, and *United States v. Duhon*, a District Court decision we anticipate will receive considerable attention in the future.

The United States Supreme Court has jurisdictional authority in all states and federal circuits. Many cases heard by this court concern alleged violations of constitutional rights. Decisions of the Supreme Court often serve to establish the minimum degree of rights afforded by the United States Constitution. No state can offer fewer rights than those specified by the Constitution (as interpreted by the United States Supreme Court). By establishing this minimum, however, the United States Supreme Court in no way bars states from offering *more* protection than that minimally required by the Constitution. In other words, when the United State Supreme Court establishes a minimum level of a constitutional right, states are free to offer more rights than required, but never less.

Most appellate decisions are made by panels of judges. In some cases, opinions are shared by all judges hearing the case, and the ruling is a unanimous one. In other cases, judges view aspects of the case differently, and the ruling represents the opinion of the majority of judges who heard the case. The majority opinion is controlling law. In some cases, judges who agree with the majority decision offer a separate concurring opinion to more clearly articulate their own views. Those who disagree with the majority sometimes write dissenting opinions that explain why they would have reached a different ruling.

In this book, we have included excerpts from majority, concurring, and dissenting opinions. We believe both the prevailing and dissenting opinions provide insight for the clinician about how courts think about psycholegal issues.

All the decisions presented in this book were heard in federal courts. District court decisions have standing only in the trial court, and circuit appellate decisions are controlling only in that circuit, although either may be cited for their persuasive authority. Decisions of the United States Supreme Court are binding in all jurisdictions, although states may offer more protections than those determined to be minimally required by the Constitution.

Section 1

Standards of Competency

Introduction to Section 1

Cases

Implications for Examiners

Introduction to Section 1

The cases presented in this section concern basic considerations about what constitutes competency to stand trial. Definitions and language have evolved over years, but the essence of competency doctrine (that it is unfair to try an incompetent defendant) has remained unchanged for centuries. A late 19th-century case, *Youtsey v. United States* (1899) traces the roots of how courts have construed the unfairness of trying incompetent defendants. The court in *Youtsey* provided a detailed analysis of early American and English law concerning standards of competency. The reader should be aware that in many early cases like *Youtsey*, the terms "competency" and "sanity" were used interchangeably.

Dusky v. United States (1960) is the United States Supreme Court case that provides the underpinning of most legal analysis of competency to stand trial. In *Dusky*, the Supreme Court established that competency entails a test of whether the defendant has sufficient present ability to consult with counsel with a reasonable degree of rational understanding and whether the defendant has a rational as well as factual understanding of the proceedings. Despite *Dusky's* importance, the Supreme Court's ruling constitutes less than two pages. To more clearly present the issues addressed in *Dusky*, we have added passages from the appellate court reviews published before and after the Supreme Court decision.

Whereas *Dusky* articulated the standard for competency, *Wieter v. Settle* (1961) provides guidance in its application. The decision in *Wieter* intimates that the criteria for competency are not difficult to attain and that most mentally ill defendants are likely able to meet them. The court even provided eight guidelines defining the minimal abilities necessary for competency. Although it is a district court case, *Wieter* is often cited for its analysis of what defendants need to be able to do to proceed.

Youtsey v. United States

97 F. 937 (6th Cir., 1899)

Facts[1]

The defendant was charged with six counts of fraud after converting approximately $15,000 of bank notes to his own use "without the knowledge or consent of the directors or the exchange committee." The defense claimed Youtsey had epilepsy to the extent "that the excitement and strain of a prolonged trial might induce another epileptic attack." Three physicians claimed Youtsey was unable to participate appropriately, having substantial impairment in judgment and memory. The defense requested a continuance for a number of reasons, including an opportunity to examine the competency of the defendant. The trial judge refused to grant the continuance.

Issue

Given a request for continuance to examine competency of a defendant, is the trial judge required to respond to the request?

Holding

Yes. The trial judge should have adopted some method of examining the competence of the defendant to proceed prior to putting him on trial.

Analysis

By a review of American and English law, the appellate court determined it is a violation of due process of law to try an incompetent defendant: "It is fundamental that an insane person can neither plead to an arraignment, be subjected to a trial, or, after trial, receive judgment, or, after judgment, undergo punishment." The trial court had broad latitude in addressing the issue of com-

---

[1] The facts of the case are not provided in the appellate decision and have been taken from trial transcripts; 91 F. 864 (1898).

petency, either by independent consideration or by subjecting the matter to the trial jury; nevertheless, some judicial response to the motion for continuance due to incompetency was required. Failure of the trial court to dispose of that issue requires a reversal of conviction and re-trial, if indicated.

Edited Excerpts[2]

YOUTSEY v. UNITED STATES

Circuit Court of Appeals, Sixth Circuit

97 F. 937

November 13, 1899

In Error to the Circuit Court of the United States for the District of Kentucky

Before Lurton, Circuit Judge, and Severens, and Clark, District Judges

Lurton, Circuit Judge

The primal question which confronts the court arises upon the objection interposed by counsel for the plaintiff in error to a trial of the accused on account of his then nonsane mind and memory. So far as this application and motion for a continuance were based upon the fact that the prisoner was a confirmed epileptic, and that his counsel and medical advisers apprehended that the excitement and strain of a prolonged trial

> **It is fundamental that an insane person can neither plead to an arraignment, be subjected to a trial, or, after trial, receive judgment, or, after judgment, undergo punishment.**

might induce another epileptic attack, it was addressed to the enlightened humanity and sound discretion of the lower court. The application, in that aspect, did not show any present inability to attend the trial, and promised no hope that any future trial would be attended by any less risk to the health or life of the accused. Under such circumstances, it was no abuse of discretion to proceed with the trial.

---

[2] Readers are advised to quote only from the original published cases. See pages vii-viii.

But the petition of the counsel involved much more than a mere continuance on account of the physical condition of the defendant. In substance and legal effect, it also presented an issue of present insanity as a bar to any trial while that condition continued, and prayed a continuance for that reason, also. The statutes of the United States present no mode for the presentation and trial of an issue of present insanity, when presented in bar of an arraignment, trial, judgment, or execution, and we must look to the common law for guidance in practice.

It is fundamental that an insane person can neither plead to an arraignment, be subjected to a trial, or, after trial, receive judgment, or, after judgment, undergo punishment. "If a man in his sound memory commits a capital offense, and before his arraignment he becomes absolutely mad, he ought not by law to be arraigned during such frenzy, but be remitted to prison until that incapacity be removed. The reason is, because he cannot advisedly plead to the indictment. And if such person of nonsane memory after his plea, and before his trial, become of nonsane memory, he shall not be tried; or, if, after his trial, he becomes of nonsane memory, he shall not receive judgment, or, if after judgment he becomes of nonsane memory, his execution shall be spared; for were he of sound memory, he might allege somewhat in stay of judgment or execution" (*1 Hale, P.C.*).

In [*Reg. v. Berry*] a deaf mute was put on his trial. The trial court put two questions to the jury: First, whether they found the prisoner guilty on the indictment; secondly, whether, in their opinion, the prisoner was capable of understanding, and had understood, the nature of the proceedings. The verdict was, "Guilty," but that the defendant was not capable of understanding, "and, as a fact, has not understood, the nature of the proceedings." Judgment was reserved until a case could be submitted to the queen's bench division. There the conviction was quashed. [In reviewing this case, an English jurist] said: "Further, I believe it to have been the law from the earliest times that if it be found, at the trial of a prisoner, that he cannot understand the proceedings, the judge ought to discharge the jury and put an end to the trial, or order a verdict of not guilty. The jury here have found the prisoner incapable of understanding, and it needs no argument to show that under such circumstances he ought not to be convicted."

> *If it appears after arraignment, and before trial, that the prisoner is probably not capable of making a rational defense, the proceedings should stop until the sanity of the prisoner is determined or restored.*

If it appears after arraignment, and before trial, that the prisoner is probably not capable of making a rational defense, the proceedings should stop until the sanity of the prisoner is determined or restored. Such an issue, when presented, goes to the fundamental right of the court to try the main issue, "Not guilty." If present insanity does not appear until the trial has begun, the court may submit the objection to the jury along with the principal issue, requiring a special verdict as to the competency of the defendant to understand the proceeding and intelligently defend himself. But, if the jury finds insanity to exist, a verdict upon the issue of not guilty should be quashed. It is not "due process of law" to subject an insane person to trial upon an indictment involving liberty or life. If the time when such an issue is presented be not vital, for a still stronger reason the mode in which the objection is urged is still less of the substance of the matter.

Youtsey was a "confirmed epileptic," and he had suffered a severe attack of epilepsy since the last continuance. To add to the *prima facie*[3] case, the affidavits of three physicians were presented, all of whom state that the plaintiff in error is a confirmed epileptic, and that the effect of the disease is to weaken the mind and memory. Dr. Charles Kearns averred that: "As a result of his numerous attacks of epilepsy, his memory and judgment have become permanently impaired; that his memory is not reliable as to ordinary occurrences of the past; and that, in the judgment of this affiant, he is not in a condition to testify in behalf of himself as to business and other transactions in which he has been engaged."

In further support of the application for a continuance, the petition invoked an investigation, and expressed the desire of counsel: "To submit the mental and physical condition of the defendant to this court for such examination by competent physicians and otherwise as

> It is not "due process of law" to subject an insane person to trial upon an indictment involving liberty or life.

the court may deem best to make, in order to determine whether the defendant should be subjected to a trial of this cause at this term."

The *prima facie* showing made by the affidavit of counsel and physicians was that the defendant's mind and memory, as a consequence of epileptic attacks, had become so impaired as that he was unable to advise his counsel as to his defense, or recall transactions which ought to have been within his knowledge, and could not "remember transactions from day to day," and that he was unable, in consequence of his impaired mind and memory, to testify for himself. This *prima facie* showing was made by persons of

---

[3] *prima facie.* Sufficiently based upon the minimum evidence required.

weight and respectability, and upon that showing the court was asked to make such examination and inquiry as would further tend to throw light upon the question of the fitness of the defendant to be put on his trial at that term of the court.

It is said, touching the manner of proceeding when present insanity is objected: "But because there may be great fraud in this matter, yet, if the crime be notorious, as treason or murder, the judge, before such respite of trial or judgment, may do well to impanel a jury to inquire *ex officio*[4] touching such insanity, and whether it be real or counterfeit" (*1 Hale, P.C.*).

In *Frith's Case*, the court, upon the objection being urged when Frith was about to be arraigned, directed a special jury to be impaneled to try the question of the fitness of the accused to be tried. But the defendant had no absolute right to a trial by jury of such a preliminary question. The most that can be inferred from the common-law authorities is that the judge may, if he has doubts, call to his assistance the aid of a jury, and submit the matter to them, and that this has been the usual practice. The mode of trial is one which addresses itself to the sound discretion of the court when the objection is made after verdict and sentence. We see no reason or authority for a different rule when the objection is made in bar of a trial.

Having the right to exercise its discretion as to the mode in which the court should investigate the mental capacity of the accused to understand the proceedings against him, and rationally advise with his counsel as to his defense, we are confronted with the question as to whether the court in any way investigated and decided the issue thus tendered by the counsel for the accused. Undoubtedly the court was bound to entertain the objection and dispose of it in some way. It is suggested that the court did so by personal inspection, and in that way satisfied itself of the competency of the accused to rationally conduct his defense.

In *People v. McElvaine*, counsel for McElvaine, after pleading "Not guilty," tendered an oral plea to the effect that the prisoner was insane, and not a fit subject for trial, and requested the court to appoint a commission under the statute to examine and report on the issue. This was denied by the court upon the

> **But because there may be great fraud in this matter, yet, if the crime be notorious, as treason or murder, the judge, before such respite of trial or judgment, may do well to impanel a jury to inquire ex officio touching such insanity, and whether it be real or counterfeit.**

ground that there was nothing in the case "from which it ap-

---

[4] *ex officio.* Officially.

peared that the defendant was then insane." McElvaine was put on his trial and convicted. One of the defenses was insanity at the time of the commission of the offense. The New York court of appeals held there was no error in denying the appointment of a statutory commission, [because]: "It had previously tried the defendant for the same crime, and had heard the evidence adduced by the defendant to support the plea of insanity. It was familiar with the appearance and conduct of the prisoner during the period of that trial, and had sufficient grounds before it to judge as to the probability of his present sanity. It thus had the prisoner before it, and witnessed his actions and manner, and had access to the information acquired by the officers of the court through their daily contact and communication with the defendant during the time of the imprisonment; and it is hardly possible that the defendant could have manifested symptoms of his insanity which would not have been discovered by, or be communicated, to the court. *There was no pretense that there had been any change in his mental condition since the previous trial, and no proof of any insanity whatever was given to support the demand for an inquisition.*" [The italics are in *Youtsey*.]

> **I came to the conclusion that the prisoner knew where he was, what he was here for, and what was being done (cited from Youtsey's trial judge).**

The case of *Webber v. [Commonwealth of Pennsylvania]* has been much relied upon by counsel for the government as sustaining their contention that this court should infer, on this record, that the trial court disposed of the issue of present insanity by inspection and on information derived from other sources satisfactory to itself. In Webber's case, his counsel filed what the report describes as "a formal suggestion" of the present insanity of the defendant, and asked that a jury be impaneled to try whether such fact be true or not, so that the court might take action under a statute of the state providing for the confinement of insane persons under indictment. This suggestion was objected to by the counsel for the state, and defendant offered to support same by affidavits and witnesses. The court declined to hear the evidence, denied the motion, and put the prisoner on his trial; one of his defenses being insanity at the time of the commission of the offense. But here the analogy between that cause and the one before us ends. It appeared on the record that the trial judge did hear, consider, and determine the issue, though he declined to hear the evidence offered in support thereof, and denied a special jury to hear the question. The trial judge inserted in the record his reasons for his action; saying, among other things, that: "Nearly two hours was consumed in the argument and consideration of the motion, during which time I had the opportunity of observing the appearance and conduct of the prisoner, and the attention he gave to the proceedings. I had also the benefit of the information of the physician of the prison and others to assist me in coming to that sound judgment which it was my duty to exercise. Giving the matter the due consideration to which it was entitled, I came to the conclusion that the prisoner knew where he was, what he was here for, and what was being done."

The supreme court of Pennsylvania, upon a consideration of the whole facts and law, held that the right of the accused to a preliminary trial by jury of the question of present insanity, in bar of a trial upon the merits of an indictment, was not an absolute one. As to the practice, the court said: "The question principally discussed in this case is a novel one. It does not appear to have ever been determined or even presented to this court before. Briefly stated, it is this: Whether a defendant in a criminal case, who alleges his insanity at the time of arraignment, is entitled, as a matter of legal right, to have a separate, independent, and preliminary trial of that question by a jury specially impaneled for the purpose. We have examined with much care the various authorities cited in the very able and exhaustive argument of the learned counsel for the plaintiff in error, and we find that in all of them the inquest was directed generally by the court of its own motion, sometimes at the instance of the attorney general, but always in cases where the appearance and the actions or the prisoner were such as to manifestly indicate a condition of insanity, either real or simulated."

Having had the question tried and considered by the trial judge in the manner stated, and then by the jury along with the principal issue, the supreme court held that there had been no abuse of the discretion of the court in refusing a preliminary inquiry, and that there was no reason for reversing the cause for such a preliminary trial. The contrast between the proceedings in that case and those in the court below is quite striking. The fact that the trial court gave consideration to the issue of present insanity, and determined it by personal inspection, aided by the counsel, opinion, and advice of the jail physician "and others," and that it also submitted to the jury the question of the present sanity of the accused, appeared affirmatively upon the record in the *Webber* appeal. The record before us is silent as to how the court satisfied itself of the sanity of the accused, in the face of the showing made by the petition and accompanying affidavits, or whether the objection was entertained and decided in any way. The issue presented by the petition and motion thereon for a continuance involved the substantial rights of the accused. If the petition truthfully described the then condition of the mind and memory of the plaintiff in error, grave doubt must arise as to whether he was a fit subject for trial.

Assuming, as we shall, that no duty rested upon the court to impanel a jury to inquire whether the accused [was] in truth incapable of understanding the proceedings, and intelligently advising with his counsel as to his defense, and that it was optional with the court to call a jury, or to resort to any other special mode of aiding his judgment, it was nevertheless his duty to consider and determine the matter judicially; and the record should show affirmatively that upon this issue there has been the exercise of judicial judgment and discretion. Whatever the court's judicial discretion as to the mode of hearing and deciding, we entertain no doubt but that it was error to refuse altogether to entertain the objection; and this, we think, is the only justifiable inference which can legitimately be drawn from the order denying a continuance, the record being otherwise silent as to the disposition of this question. However wide the discretion of a trial court in respect to the mode of disposing of such an issue as that now involved, if the court has refused altogether to consider, hear, and determine in any way an issue of present insanity, when properly presented as a bar to a trial, there has been no exercise of discretion, and the action of the court is subject to review.

Epilepsy is a progressive disease, and its effect upon the mind and memory is progressive. There was evidence strongly tending to show that the memory and mind of accused shortly before and during the trial were impaired, and rendering it doubtful whether the accused was capable of appreciating his situation, and of intelligently advising his counsel as to his defense, if any he had. This evidence indicated that the disease had progressed, and with it the impairment of mind and memory. We think the learned trial judge should have adopted some method of satisfying himself that the accused was able to rationally defend himself, before putting him on trial under the plea of not guilty. For this error we are constrained to reverse the case, with directions that a new trial be awarded, and that before such trial some mode, in the discretion of the court, be adopted for a thorough investigation of the sanity of the accused.

Dusky v. United States

362 U.S. 402 (1960)

Facts

Defendant Milton Dusky was arrested and charged with kidnapping and raping a 15-year-old girl. Prior to trial, Dusky was evaluated at the U.S. Medical Center for Federal Prisoners in Springfield, Missouri, to determine if he was competent to proceed to trial. A competency hearing was held, at which a psychiatrist testified that because of severe mental illness, Dusky evidenced confused thinking, was unable to distinguish reality from unreality, was unable to properly understand the proceedings against him, and was unable to adequately assist counsel in his defense. The psychiatrist also testified that Dusky was oriented to time, place, and person. The district court judge declared Dusky competent, stating, "Since he is oriented as to time, place, and person, since he, in my opinion based on the limited evidence that has been presented so far, is able to assist counsel in his own defense, then it will be concluded that he is mentally competent to stand trial."

Procedural History

Dusky was subsequently tried and convicted. Dusky appealed to the Court of Appeals for the Eighth Circuit contending that the trial judge was in error in concluding Dusky was competent in the face of expert testimony to the contrary. The Eighth Circuit affirmed the judgment of conviction. Dusky appealed to the United States Supreme Court.

Issue

What is the test for determining whether a defendant is competent to stand trial?

Holding

The test for determining a defendant's competency to stand trial is "whether he has sufficient present ability to consult with his lawyer with a reasonable degree of rational understanding -

and whether he has a rational as well as factual understanding of the proceedings against him."

Analysis

It is fundamentally unfair to try someone for an offense unless the person is able to understand the pending charges and is able to participate in the development or presentation of a defense. It is not enough for the district court to find that the defendant is oriented to time and place and has some recollection of the events in question. The test must be whether the defendant has sufficient present ability to consult with his lawyer with a reasonable degree of rational understanding and whether he has a rational as well as factual understanding of the proceedings against him.

Edited Excerpts[1]

Eighth Circuit (1st Appeal)

Milton R. Dusky, Appellant, v. United States of America, Appellee

271 F.2d 385

November 6, 1959

Before Sanborn, Woodrough, and Matthes, Circuit Judges

Sanborn, Circuit Judge

This is an appeal from a judgment and sentence of imprisonment based upon the verdict of a jury finding the defendant, Milton R. Dusky, guilty under an indictment returned September 10, 1958, charging him with having, on or about August 19, 1958, unlawfully transported in interstate commerce from Johnson County, Kansas, to Ruskin Heights, Missouri, a certain girl who had been unlawfully decoyed, kidnapped, and carried away.

Broadly stated, the main contentions of the defendant are, in substance, that the court committed reversible error (1) in finding him mentally competent to stand trial; (2) in denying his motion, made at the close of the evidence at the trial, for a directed verdict of acquittal, and in submitting the issue of his sanity to the jury; and (3) in instructing the jury on that issue.

---

[1] Readers are advised to quote only from the original published cases. See pages vii-viii.

Upon his arraignment on September 12, 1958, the defendant entered a plea of not guilty. At the suggestion of his counsel that there was a question of the defendant's mental competency to stand trial and that there might be a question whether he could be found mentally responsible for the crime charged against him, the court, pursuant to [federal statute], ordered the defendant committed to the United States Medical Center for Federal Prisoners at Springfield, Missouri, for examination as to his mental competency to stand trial, and, in addition, "to determine, insofar as possible, whether, on August 19, 1958, the defendant was possessed of sufficient mental and moral faculties as to be capable of distinguishing between right and wrong and to be conscious of the nature of the acts which he was then doing or committing."

The court had before it a detailed report of a Neuropsychiatric Examination of the defendant. This report was dated October 30, 1958, and was signed by Doctor L. Moreau, Staff Psychiatrist at Medical Center. On the last page of the report appears the following: "He is oriented as to time, place, and person. He denies complete memory of the events of the day of the alleged offense. He gives the

> *The evidence of the psychiatrists as to the competency of the defendant to stand trial was not unequivocal, and it was not shown that he was unable to understand the proceedings against him.*

impression clinically of being of approximately average intelligence. His responses to the abstractions tests indicate approximately normal capacity for abstract thinking."

The only witness testifying at the hearing was Doctor Sturgell, whose testimony was in substantial conformity with the reports in evidence. He explained the statement in Doctor Moreau's report that the defendant was oriented as to time, place, and person. Doctor Sturgell also expressed the opinion that the defendant understood what he was charged with, knew that if there was a trial it would be before a judge and jury, knew that if found guilty he could be punished, and knew who his attorney was and that it was his duty to protect the defendant's rights. It appeared from Doctor Sturgell's testimony also that the defendant had been able to furnish, with substantial accuracy, information as to his past history and as to at least some of the events leading up to the occurrence upon which the indictment was based. The Doctor expressed the opinion that the defendant would be unable properly to assist his attorney in his defense "because I do not think that he can properly interpret the meaning of the things that have happened. I don't think he can convey full knowledge of his actual circumstances due to an inability to interpret reality from unreality, to suspicions of what is going on, to confused thinking, which is part of his mental illness." The Doctor also testified that the defendant "would be able to tell his attorney of the events, as he recalls them, as interpreted by the thinking which is directly connected with his mental illness," which could result in a false factual statement to his attorney.

Doctor Sturgell stated that the defendant, who - the report of Neuropsychiatric Examination dated October 30, 1958, showed - had said he drank two pints of vodka during the night before the acts of August 19, 1958, were committed, and continued to drink heavily the following day, could have been drunk, and so unable to remember the crucial events of that day. There was other testimony by the Doctor in support of his views that the mental illness of the defendant would or could disable him from adequately assisting his counsel in his defense, but enough has been said to indicate the views of the Psychiatric Staff of the Medical Center as to the mental competency of the defendant to stand trial.

The District Judge, at the conclusion of the hearing, decided that the defendant had sufficient mental competency to stand trial, saying: "That is not in any way saying, gentlemen, that he is responsible, as not being mentally incompetent, for the offense for which he is being tried. It is simply in the narrow test [of the federal statute] that is used. Since he is oriented as to time and place and person, since he, in my opinion based on the limited evidence that has been presented so far, is able to assist counsel in his own defense, then it will be concluded that he is mentally competent to stand trial and will be retained here until the case is set for trial."

Defendant's counsel then made the following statement: "Your Honor, may the record show my objection and exception to the Court's ruling in view of the undisputed testimony of the Government's witness, the psychiatrist, the Government psychiatrist, that he (the defendant) is not properly able to assist in his defense and I, as his attorney, have reached that same conclusion, although I do not feel, as his attorney, that I should take the witness stand and

> *How much mental capacity or alertness a defendant must have to be able to assist his counsel in a case where the defense is insanity, is, we think, a question of fact for the trial court.*

be sworn and offer evidence in that regard. I make this statement as a lawyer to the Court and I believe that the man is not properly able to assist his counsel in his defense and should not be tried at this time."

The Government's evidence with respect to the events which gave rise to the indictment was uncontradicted. The victim of the kidnapping was a high school girl 15 years of age at the time. She lived with her parents in Ruskin Heights, a suburb of Kansas City, Missouri. On August 19, 1958, about noon, while she was walking to a drug store in Ruskin Heights to have lunch with a friend, the defendant with two boys - Leonard Dischart, 14 years of age, and Richard Nixon, 16 years of age - drove up in the defendant's automobile and gave her a ride to the drug store. She was an acquaintance of Nixon. After leaving her, they went down to the "Wheel-Inn Drive-In," in Ruskin Heights, where they had a discussion about taking the girl out for the purpose of having sexual intercourse with her. They were all drinking vodka. After that, they went back to the drug store, and there, or near there, decoyed her into the automobile under the pretext of taking her home and also to see some girl she knew. She was driven to a back road in Kansas, where she was forcibly undressed and raped by the two boys, and where the defendant attempted to rape her. After these happenings, the girl was permitted to put her clothing on, and was driven by the defendant, in his car, accompanied by the boys, back to Ruskin Heights, Missouri. The car stopped at the "Wheel-Inn Drive-In," where the girl, who was permitted to get out of the car for a drink of water, ran into the back room of the Drive-In and told a Mr. Delair, whom she knew, that she had been raped. Thereupon the defendant and the two boys drove away.

The defense at the trial was insanity. Under the evidence of the Government, no other defense would seem to have been available to the defendant. He and Dischart were arrested in the evening of August 20, 1958, under a warrant. Upon being advised at that time that the charge was kidnapping, the defendant said: "That is a pretty serious charge, isn't it?" Upon being told it referred to the "girl that you all picked up the other morning out in Ruskin Heights," the defendant said: "That wasn't a kidnapping. She got in the car voluntarily."

Charles W. Harris, Field Director for the American Red Cross, in the Veterans Administration Regional Office in Kansas City, Missouri, testified relative to the defendant's applications to the Red Cross for monetary assistance, and help with family problems and hospitalization. Harris testified that he had received a letter from the defendant from the Medical Center, dated November 1, 1958, which contained this language: "I am writing to let you know that the doctors here at the Medical Center have found me incompetent. Will this affect my compensation rating? It appears to me it should be increased. Would you please write and advise me on this matter."

It seems clear to us that, under [federal statute], the duty and responsibility of determining whether a defendant who has a mental illness or defect is or is not competent to stand trial is that of the trial court, and that his determination in that regard cannot be set aside on review unless clearly arbitrary or unwarranted.

The evidence of the psychiatrists as to the competency of the defendant to stand trial was not unequivocal, and it was not shown that he was unable to understand the proceedings against him. How much mental capacity or alertness a defendant must have to be able to assist his counsel in a case where the defense is insanity, is, we think, a question of fact for the trial court. This Court has consistently adhered to the policy of not requiring a trial judge to believe evidence which he finds unconvincing, and of declining to substitute its judgment for his upon issues which it is his function to determine. We are satisfied that the trial court did not commit reversible error in requiring the defendant to go to trial despite the opinion of the psychiatric staff of the Medical Center. Needless to say, expert opinion rises no higher than the reasons upon which it is based, and is not binding upon the trier of the facts.

> **Needless to say, expert opinion rises no higher than the reasons upon which it is based, and is not binding upon the trier of the facts.**

In our opinion, it was the duty and responsibility of the trial court to determine whether the defendant was competent to stand trial, and it was for the jury to decide whether, under the evidence, there was a reasonable doubt as to the defendant's sanity at the time the offense was committed. We think that nothing occurred at the trial which would justify this Court in reversing the judgment appealed from.

Supreme Court

Dusky v. United States

On petition for writ of certiorari to the United States Court of Appeals for the Eighth Circuit

362 U.S. 402

April 18, 1960

per curiam[2]

Upon consideration of the entire record we agree with the Solicitor General that "the record in this case does not sufficiently

---

[2] *per curiam.* By the court, no single opinion writer identified.

support the findings of competency to stand trial," for to support those findings under [federal statute] the district judge "would need more information than this record presents." We also agree with the suggestion of the Solicitor General that it is not enough for the district judge to find that "the defendant is oriented to time and place and has some recollection of events," but that the "test must be whether he has sufficient present ability to consult with his lawyer with a reasonable degree of rational understanding - and whether he has a rational as well as factual understanding of the proceedings against him."

In view of the doubts and ambiguities regarding the legal significance of the psychiatric testimony in this case and the resulting difficulties of retrospectively determining the petitioner's competency as of more than a year ago, we reverse the judgment of the Court of Appeals affirming the judgment of conviction, and remand the case to the District Court for a new hearing to ascertain petitioner's present competency to stand trial, and for a new trial if petitioner is found competent.

> *The test must be whether he has sufficient present ability to consult with his lawyer with a reasonable degree of rational understanding and whether he has a rational as well as factual understanding of the proceedings against him.*

Eighth Circuit (2d Appeal)

Milton R. Dusky, Appellant, v. United States of America, Appellee

United States Court of Appeals, Eighth Circuit

295 F.2d 743

November 3, 1961

Before Vogel and Blackmun, Circuit Judges, and Beck, District Judge

Blackmun, Circuit Judge

The required new hearing to ascertain the defendant's competency to stand trial was held October 3, 1960, this time before the Honorable Albert A. Ridge, then Chief Judge of the United States District Court for the Western District of Missouri. Dr. John Kendall Dickinson, a staff psychiatrist at the Springfield Medical Center, whose testimony at the subsequent trial is hereinafter described, and Dr. Joseph C. Sturgell, chief of the psychiatric staff there, both testified at that hearing. Their testimony and the June 1960 written report of the Center's staff were to the effect, specifically, that the defendant was then oriented as to time, place, and person; that he had some recollection of the events surrounding the offense with which he was charged; that he had present ability to consult with his lawyer with a reasonable degree of rational understanding; that he had a rational as well as a factual understanding of the proceedings in court against him; and that, generally, he was competent to stand trial. Defense counsel expressed his confidence in the psychiatrists and acknowledged to the court that he was not then experiencing the difficulty in consulting and working with his client which he had encountered at the time of the first trial. It will be noted that the evidence produced at this hearing was along the exact lines of the test set forth by the Supreme Court. Judge Ridge accordingly found that the defendant was competent to stand trial.

Wieter v. Settle

193 F. Supp. 318 (W.D. Mo., 1961)

Facts

Kenneth Jerome Wieter was taken into custody by agents of the Federal Bureau of Investigation on an arrest warrant issued for a misdemeanor offense. He was evaluated by a local psychiatrist and was adjudicated mentally incompetent and incapable of understanding the proceedings against him or properly assisting in his own defense. As a result of this adjudication, he was committed to the custody of the Attorney General for hospitalization and care until such time that he became mentally competent to stand trial or "until the pending charges against him [were] disposed of according to law." He was subsequently confined for 18 months for treatment to restore competency. After being in custody for over 19 months on misdemeanor charges, Wieter petitioned for a writ of *habeas corpus*.[1]

Issue

Is a defendant who is charged with a misdemeanor, and who has been committed to a medical center for 18 months on the grounds of incompetency, entitled to release on *habeas corpus* on the grounds that further prosecution is no longer probable?

Holding

Yes. It is improper to detain someone charged with a misdemeanor for competency restoration treatment, if prosecution is no longer probable.

Analysis

Wieter factually established a legal right to release from federal criminal custody when further prosecution is no longer probable (i.e., further federal prosecution had probably been "irretrievably frustrated"). The court noted that "the propriety of a

---

[1] writ of *habeas corpus*. A request to come before the court to ask for release from custody.

criminal pretrial commitment to a special institution for the criminally insane should turn on the existence of a *bona fide* criminal accusation." Additionally, the court provided guidelines establishing minimal abilities necessary for competency.

Edited Excerpts[2]

Kenneth Jerome Wieter, Petitioner, v. Dr. R. O. Settle, Warden, United States Medical Center, Springfield, Missouri, Respondent

United States District Court for the Western District of Missouri, Western Division

193 F. Supp. 318

April 13, 1961

Ridge, Chief Judge

Petitioner has been confined in the Medical Center for Federal Prisoners, at Springfield, Missouri, for over 15 months, as a consequence of an order of the United States District Court for the Southern District of California [on a misdemeanor charge]. At a hearing in this Court on petition for writ of *habeas corpus*, these salient facts were established: September 28, 1959, petitioner was taken into custody by members of the Federal Bureau of Investigation, on warrant for his arrest issued on the complaint. On October 8, 1959, he was examined by a local psychiatrist appointed by the United States District Court for the Southern District of California, who made a report to that Court on October 16, 1959. [On] November 2, 1959, a hearing was held in the above District Court, at the conclusion of which that Court found petitioner to be mentally incompetent and incapable of understanding the proceedings against him or properly assisting in his own defense. As a result, petitioner was committed to the custody of the Attorney General "for hospitalization and care until such time as the defendant shall be mentally competent to stand trial or until the pending charges against him are disposed of according to law." It was directed that he be confined in the Medical Center under that order, on January 8, 1960, by the Director of the Bureau of Prisons. He was accordingly placed in the custody of respondent on January 20, 1960.

---

[2] Readers are advised to quote only from the original published cases. See pages vii-viii.

At the time neuropsychiatric examinations were made, on March 17, 1960 and at the time of petitioner's appearance before the Neuropsychiatric Staff of the Medical Center on April 13, 1960, and November 16, 1960, it appears from Staff Reports that petitioner was well oriented in the three spheres, of places, persons, and things; without perceptible abnormalities of hallucinations or delusions; seemingly, with intelligence in the average

> *Petitioner had then been in the custody of Government authorities for more than any term of confinement that might have been meted out on a finding of guilt of the misdemeanor charge.*

range, although he appeared to be confused in his thought processes, with a tendency to lose emotional control when talking about his present and past offenses and his hospitalization, and retreated into autistic hyper-religious ideations; and that petitioner's judgment appeared to be severely diminished around the incidents in his life as to which he seems unable to integrate his role as a causative factor in determining his situation. The original diagnosis of petitioner made on April 17, 1960, was: "Schizophrenic reaction, paranoid type, in partial and tenuous remission, manifested by hyper-religiosity, decreased self-control, life history of social and occupational instability, excessive dependency on institutional living, excessive suspiciousness, and grandiose and persecutory ideas."

At the last-above-mentioned date, it should be noted that petitioner had then been in the custody of Government authorities, under arrest status, for more than any term of confinement that might have been meted out on a finding of guilt of the misdemeanor charge, for which petitioner was originally taken into custody. But for the *habeas corpus* proceeding commenced in this Court on February 13, 1961, petitioner would, in all probability, not have been released from such custody, under the commitment on which he was confined in the Medical Center, until sometime in May, next. Such release would have been for return to his committing Court to stand trial on the charge there made against him.

The issue raised and presented in the instant *habeas corpus* proceeding is a classic example of similar matters, recurrently arising and presented to this District Court by virtue of commitments of persons arrested but not convicted of any federal offense, as authorized by [federal statute]. In many such cases this Court is confronted with a conclusion of the Neuropsychiatric Staff of the Medical Center, that the petitioner, considered from psychiatric discipline, is unable to rationally understand the nature of the criminal proceedings pending against him and is unable to rationally cooperate with his counsel in defense thereto. However, when some such persons personally appear before this District Court in a *habeas corpus* proceeding it is evident from legal concepts that they, in all probability, are possessed of mental faculties that would sanction their right to stand trial on the charge made against them; and that this Court, in failing to recognize and so adjudicate that fact, would be on the threshold of cooperatively denying some such persons the right to a "speedy" trial as commanded by the Sixth Amendment[3] to the Constitution of the United States. In the statement of that proposition, no intendment to disparage any conclusion of the Neuropsychiatric Staff of the Medical Center for Federal Prisoners, at Springfield, Missouri, should be inferred or understood. The incongruity in that situation arises from a long-standing, recognizable inability to effect a complete reconciliation between the medical tests of "mental illness" that disqualifies a person under the psychiatric discipline as being unable to stand trial on the charge of law violation; and, the legal tests of criminal responsibility fashioned in ancient standards of criminal procedure which time and human experience have proved adequate in protection of individual human rights.

Though psychiatry discipline may term it hyperbole, nevertheless, when it is evidentially made to appear in a *habeas corpus* proceeding by a person under arrest status, confined pursuant to [federal statute]: (1) that he has mental capacity to appreciate his presence in relation to time, place, and things; (2) that his elementary mental processes are such that he apprehends (i.e., seizes and grasps with what mind he has) that he is in a Court of Justice, charged with a criminal offense; (3) that there is a Judge on the Bench; (4) a Prosecutor present who will try to convict him of a criminal charge; (5) that he has a lawyer (self-employed or Court-appointed) who will undertake to defend him against that charge; (6) that he will be expected to tell his lawyer the circumstances, to the best of his mental ability (whether colored or not by mental aberration), the facts surrounding him at the time and place where the law violation is alleged to have been committed; (7) that there is, or will be, a jury present to pass upon evidence adduced as to his guilt or innocence of such charge; and (8) he has memory sufficient to relate those things in his own personal manner. [S]uch a person, from a consideration of legal standards, should be considered mentally competent to stand trial under criminal procedure, lawfully enacted. At that time, in criminal procedure, such a person is not in the position of being evaluated as capable, or incapable, of knowing right from wrong; or as being

---

[3] Sixth Amendment. See Appendix B (pp. 261-262).

"mentally ill" or afflicted with "mental disease" from psychiatric standards so that he may, psychiatrically, be concluded as mentally unable to rationally understand the proceedings against him and cooperate with counsel in his own defense. Any such psychiatric conclusion, if arrived at, is not and cannot be legally binding. At most, it is merely opinion testimony, to be resolved by the legal finder of fact, in the same manner as is the testimony of all expert expressed conclusions. Any difference between legal and psychiatric disciplines respecting the latter proposition, arises from failure to appreciate that: "Opinion testimony is one of those practical anomalies of the law of evidence devised to help (the finder of fact) understand technical subjects on which they (would be) required to speculate or guess without some expert explanation." (Parentheses in the original.)

Petitioner in this *habeas corpus* proceeding, by evidence (testimony and written documents) established the above eight criteria to the reasonable satisfaction of this Court. All that this Court may do in such an action is to consider whether probable cause of mental competency to stand trial is established, which, in justice and within the Sixth Amendment concepts, compels that he be returned to his committing Court for a fur-

> *Opinion testimony is devised to help the finder of fact understand technical subjects on which they would be required to speculate or guess without some expert explanation.*

ther determination thereof. That such power exists in a *habeas corpus* proceeding is made manifest when the eight above-recited legal concepts are shown to exist by competent evidence and a defendant is retained in the Medical Center against his will; which latter fact is always made manifest.

It appears from the facts heretofore stated that this case is a case in which further federal prosecution has probably been "irretrievably frustrated." A misdemeanor, committed 19½ months ago, recognized by a complaint filed and arrest thereon the same date; with a commitment under [federal statute] for a period of 18 months of that time, against the will of defendant, as made manifest by the order of commitment; a situation which, in all probability, will continue, in the face of psychiatric testimony adduced by the Government that in the opinion of "The Psychiatric Staff (of the Medical Center, petitioner's) present treatment program (should) be continued for another three month period," and, the additional fact appearing that petitioner, since his confinement, has demanded trial on such charge; leads inevitably to that conclusion. Petitioner can no longer be retained in federal criminal custody.

It is so ordered.

Implications for Examiners

Although the case is over 100 years old, *Youtsey* highlights a problem that exists to this day. Simply put, courts often fall prey to the allure of diagnoses. Legal professionals who do not routinely encounter mental health issues are apt to equate the presence of certain mental health disorders with the legal construct of incompetency. Courts may be more impressed with the diagnostic label than with the presence or absence of the specific abilities necessary for an individual to competently proceed. (Unfortunately, many inexperienced examiners are similarly impressed.) Thus, it becomes the appropriate role of the expert to explain for the court the meaning of any diagnosis and the impact of a defendant's mental state on the requisite abilities.

The decision in *Dusky* underscored the importance of this distinction. In adopting a test for competency that focuses on understanding and ability, the Supreme Court established an important role for mental health experts. Clinicians will best serve the court by detailing what a defendant can and cannot do, relevant to the abilities which underlie competency.

Although statutes in most jurisdictions track the language offered by the Supreme Court in *Dusky*, some ambiguity remains, both in the meaning of the language and in its practical application. *Wieter* suggests that *Dusky* established a fairly low level of requisite ability. The judge's attempt to delineate a list of observable behavior reflects an understandable impulse to move from the abstract to the specific.

Because the standard for competency may be open to interpretation, especially by courts that equate diagnosis with incompetency, clinicians should provide a sound and detailed rationale for their opinions. Decisions regarding incompetency are solely within the purview of the court. However, courts will be best informed when guided by careful analyses of the specific, relevant abilities of the defendant, analyses that are within the purview of mental health professionals. The focus should be on providing useful data which can inform the court's decision, not on generating an opinion on the legal issue.

Section 2

Thresholds for Competency Examinations

Introduction to Section 2

Cases

Implications for Examiners

Introduction to Section 2

These cases concern when and why courts must make assessments of competency to stand trial. These issues are often predicated on whether a court had sufficient cause for concern given information about the defendant's past mental health history or any current behavior that suggests mental disorder. In *Kenner v. United States* (1960), the trial court denied a motion for a mental health examination, despite reports of the defendant's current strange behavior, because mental health examinations conducted years earlier concluded Kenner did not have an active mental disorder. By overturning a conviction delivered when Kenner may have been incompetent, the appellate court affirmed that a competent defendant is a prerequisite to a fair trial. In *Pate v. Robinson* (1966), the U.S. Supreme Court established that any concerns about competency, when raised in good faith, require the trial judge to hold a hearing on the issue. Failure to do so infringes upon the defendant's constitutional right to due process. In *Drope v. Missouri* (1975), the U.S. Supreme Court asserted that further inquiry and examination is required when there is sufficient doubt as to a defendant's competence to stand trial. Failure to do so constitutes a deprivation of due process rights to a fair trial. *Seidner v. United States* (1958) held that the issue of a defendant's competency to stand trial can be raised even after conviction and sentencing. Seidner did not believe he was mentally ill and did not want a retrospective examination of his competency at the time of trial. The court held that fundamental fairness required such an examination even over Seidner's objections.

Kenner v. United States

286 F.2d 208 (8th Cir., 1960)

Facts

John Henry Kenner was convicted and sentenced to 5 years of imprisonment. Motions for a psychiatric examination had been submitted before and during his trial. The defense attorney reported Kenner was "incoherent in speech" and not able to assist in his defense by giving "even a straight story as to the facts of the case." Upon reading a probation office report indicating that psychiatric evaluations completed 7 years previously had diagnosed Kenner only with "antisocial personality," the court denied the motion for examination. The case was heard on appeal to Court of Appeals for the Eighth Circuit after Kenner's conviction, to determine whether the trial court committed an error by denying motions requesting a competency examination prior to trial.

Issue

What type of information justifies a trial court's denial of a defendant's motion for a competency examination?

Holding

A motion made on behalf of an accused for a competency examination, made in good faith and not frivolous, must be granted.

Analysis

Federal statute required the U.S. Attorney to file a motion for a judicial determination of mental competency of the accused whenever there was reasonable cause to believe a defendant may be so mentally impaired as to be unable to understand the proceedings or to properly assist his or her attorney. In the present case, nothing in the record justified the conclusion that the motion on behalf of the appellant was frivolous or not made in good faith. Here, the psychiatric examinations, of which the court had only a probation officer's summary, had been made a number of years ago. A mental health examination was necessary in the interests of justice, as Kenner had suffered a serious brain injury and had a history of blackouts. Additionally, court-appointed counsel claimed the appellant was unable to assist in his defense. Thus, Kenner's mental competency was subject to further examination, even after sentencing.

Edited Excerpts[1]

John Henry Kenner, Appellant, v. United States of America, Appellee

United States Court of Appeals Eighth Circuit

286 F.2d 208

December 21, 1960

Before Vogel and Blackmun, Circuit Judges, and Davies, District Judge

Vogel, Circuit Judge

The appeal here is for the purpose of determining whether or not the trial court committed error in the denial of motions requesting an examination by a psychiatrist and made by appellant through his court-appointed counsel prior to trial. A motion was first made orally before the court on October 16, 1959, when appellant appeared for possible waiver of indictment. Upon reading a Probation Office report, indicating that the appellant had been examined at the Medical Center at Springfield, Missouri, and other places prior thereto, the court denied the motion. On December 4, 1959, appellant again moved for an examination, the motion taking the form of an affidavit made by counsel setting forth that in his opinion there was a definite need for a psychiatrist to determine the question of sanity. Counsel stated, in orally arguing the motion, that: "But the thing is, I have found him to be incoherent in speech. He has not been able to assist in his defense by giving me even a straight story as to the facts in the case." The motion was overruled.

It is the contention of the government that the information contained in the pre-sentence report made by a Probation Officer was sufficient basis [under federal statute] for the trial court's

---

[1] Readers are advised to quote only from the original published cases. See pages vii-viii.

denial of appellant's motion. That report indicates that in July 1952, in an Army hospital in Japan, he had an operation for the removal of bone fragments from his brain caused by a gunshot wound occurring in 1949 and that a tantalum plate was applied to the skull; that he had a history of "black-out spells"; that he was scheduled to report to the Veterans Administration Hospital in St. Louis on October 5, 1959, to determine the cause of the

> **The court therefore must cause such an examination to be made in every case, where a motion is filed that cannot be declared to be without good faith or to be frivolous.**

alleged "black-out spells." The report includes the Probation Officer's summary of the appellant's file in a Veterans Administration Regional Office in St. Louis. The summary indicated that the appellant was given a psychiatric examination while in the army in December 1952; that "His mental status was described as moderately retarded, dull. No evidence of psychosis; not insane; knew the difference between right and wrong. Diagnosis: Antisocial personality." The report also indicates that the appellant was given a psychiatric examination at the United States Army Hospital at Fort McClellan, Alabama, in May 1953; that the diagnosis was "Anti-social personality, severe, based on pathological lying, criminalism, misconduct, habitual shirker, etc. Was mentally responsible and knew the difference between right and wrong."

The only question here is: Did such information justify the trial court's denial of appellant's motion? We think it did not and that error was committed in the denial.

(Citing *Krupnick v. United States*) "The court therefore must cause such an examination to be made in every case, where a motion is filed that cannot be declared to be without good faith or to be frivolous, and where the grounds set forth thus can constitute reasonable cause to believe that the accused 'may be presently insane or otherwise so mentally incompetent as to be unable to understand the proceedings against him or properly to assist in his own defense.' "

In that case [i.e., *Krupnick*], as in the instant one, the appellant was tried and convicted subsequent to the court's denial of his motion for the examination. He would be entitled to have his sentence vacated only if it is invalid. It would not be invalid, if he was mentally competent to stand trail, in that he was at the time able to understand the proceedings against him and properly to assist in his own defense, so that his conviction did not rest on process void from insanity.

The situation here requires like result and Kenner's request for reversal must presently be refused. If he was mentally competent to stand trial at the time so as to understand the proceedings against him and to properly assist in his own defense, then his conviction was not invalid and must stand. As in *Krupnick*, appellant's mental competency is subject to a *nunc pro tunc*[2] determination.

---

[2] *nunc pro tunc* determination. Supplementing a prior determination.

Pate v. Robinson

383 U.S. 375 (1966)

Facts

In 1959, Theodore Robinson was convicted of the murder of his common-law wife. He was sentenced to imprisonment for life. It was conceded at trial that Robinson shot and killed his wife. His court-appointed counsel claimed Robinson was insane at the time of the shooting. The uncontradicted testimony of four witnesses revealed that Robinson had a long history of disturbed behavior and irrational episodes. At trial, Robinson presented as mentally alert and displayed understanding in his conversations with the trial judge. No hearing with respect to competency to stand trial was conducted.

Procedural History

The Illinois Supreme Court affirmed the conviction, rejecting the contention that Robinson had been deprived of due process. The court concluded no competency hearing had been requested, and the evidence failed to raise sufficient doubt as to Robinson's competency so as to require the court to conduct a competency hearing on its own motion. The U.S. Supreme Court denied *certiorari*.[1] Robinson then filed a petition for *habeas corpus*[2] relief in district court. The petition was denied without a hearing. The Court of Appeals for the Seventh Circuit held that Robinson was convicted in an unduly hurried trial without a fair opportunity to obtain expert psychiatric testimony and without sufficient exploration of the facts on the issue of his competency to stand trial. The Court of Appeals remanded the case to the district court with directions to hold a hearing as to whether Robinson had been denied due process by the state court's failure to conduct a hearing regarding his competency to stand trial. The U.S. Supreme Court accepted *certiorari* and held that Robinson was constitutionally entitled to have had a hearing. Given that it was too late to hold a meaningful hearing, the U.S. Supreme Court remanded the case

---

[1] *certiorari.* A means of gaining appellate review.
[2] writ of *habeas corpus.* A request to come before the court to ask for release from custody.

to the District Court with directions to discharge Robinson from custody if the state did not re-try him within a reasonable time.

Issue

When must the issue of competency be raised?

Holding

Where the evidence raises a *"bona fide* doubt" as to a defendant's competence to stand trial, and the issue is not raised by either the prosecution or defense, the judge, *sua sponte,*[3] must conduct a hearing as to the defendant's competency.

Analysis

It is well settled that the conviction of a defendant while he is legally incompetent violates due process, and state procedures must be adequate to protect this right. In this case, Robinson's constitutional rights were abridged by his failure to receive an adequate hearing on his competence to stand trial. At trial, un-contradicted testimony was introduced on Robinson's history of pronounced irrational behavior. Although his demeanor at trial might be relevant to the ultimate decision as to his competency, it was not sufficient to justify dispensing with a hearing on that very issue. The failure to observe procedures adequate to protect a defendant's right not to be tried or convicted while incompetent to stand trial deprives him of his due process right to a fair trial under the Fourteenth Amendment.[4] In its opinion, the Supreme Court also noted the difficulty of retrospectively determining competency, concluding Robinson's conviction should be vacated. The state could re-try him, if he were competent.

Edited Excerpts[5]

Frank J. Pate, Warden, Petitioner v. Theodore Robinson

Supreme Court of the United States

Certiorari to the United States Court of Appeals for the Seventh Circuit

---

[3] *sua sponte.* On the court's own initiative.

[4] Due Process Clause of the Fourteenth Amendment (Section 1). See Appendix B (p. 262).

[5] Readers are advised to quote only from the original published cases. See pages vii-viii.

383 U.S. 375

March 7, 1966

Judges: Warren, Fortas, Harlan, Brennan, Black, Stewart, Clark, White, Douglas

Mr. Justice Clark
Delivered the Opinion of the Court

In 1959 respondent Robinson was convicted of the murder of his common-law wife, Flossie May Ward, and was sentenced to imprisonment for life. Being an indigent he was defended by court-appointed counsel. It was conceded at trial that Robinson shot and killed Flossie May, but his counsel claimed that he was insane at the time of the shooting and raised the issue of his incompetence to stand trial. On writ of error to the Supreme Court of Illinois it was asserted that the trial court's rejection of these contentions deprived Robinson of due process of law under the Fourteenth Amendment. His conviction was affirmed, the court finding that no hearing on mental capacity to stand trial had been requested, that the evidence failed to raise sufficient doubt as to his competence to require the trial court to conduct a hearing on its own motion, and further that the evidence did not raise a "reasonable doubt" as to his sanity at the time of the offense. We denied *certiorari*.

Thereupon, Robinson filed this petition for *habeas corpus*, which was denied without a hearing by the United States District Court for the Northern District of Illinois. The Court of Appeals reversed, on the ground that Robinson was convicted in an unduly hurried trial without a fair opportunity to obtain expert psychiatric testimony, and without sufficient development of the facts on the issues of Robinson's insanity when he committed the homicide and his present incompetence. It remanded the case to the District Court with directions to appoint counsel for Robinson; to hold a hearing as to his sanity when he committed the alleged offense; and, if it found him to have been insane at that time, to order his release, subject to an examination into his present mental condition. The Court of Appeals directed that the District Court should also determine upon the hearing whether Robinson was denied due process by the state court's failure to conduct a hearing upon his competence to stand trial; and, if it were found his rights had been violated in this respect, that Robinson "should be ordered released, but such release may be delayed for a reasonable time to permit the State of Illinois to grant Robinson a new trial."

We have concluded that Robinson was constitutionally entitled to a hearing on the issue of his competence to stand trial. Since we do not think there could be a meaningful hearing on that issue at this late date, we direct that the District Court, after affording the State another opportunity to put Robinson to trial on its charges within a reasonable time, order him discharged. Accordingly, we affirm the decision of the Court of Appeals in this respect, except insofar as it contemplated a hearing in the District Court on Robinson's competence.

The State concedes that the conviction of an accused person while he is legally incompetent violates due process (*Bishop v. United States*), and that state procedures must be adequate to protect this right. It insists, however, that Robinson intelligently waived this issue by his failure to request a hearing on his competence at the trial; and, further, that on the basis of the evidence before the trial judge no duty rested upon him to order a hearing *sua sponte*. A determination of these claims necessitates a detailed discussion of the conduct of the trial and the evidence touching upon the question of Robinson's competence at that time.

> *The mother stated that he "had that starey look and seemed to be just a little foamy at the mouth."*

The uncontradicted testimony of four witnesses called by the defense revealed that Robinson had a long history of disturbed behavior. His mother testified that when he was between 7 and 8 years of age a brick dropped from a third floor hit Robinson on the head. "He blacked out and the blood run from his head like a faucet." Thereafter "he acted a little peculiar." The blow knocked him "cockeyed" and his mother took him to a specialist "to correct the crossness of his eyes." He also suffered headaches during his childhood, apparently stemming from the same event. His conduct became noticeably erratic about 1946 or 1947 when he was visiting his mother on a furlough from the Army. While Robinson was sitting and talking with a guest, "he jumped up and run to a bar and kicked a hole in the bar and he run up in the front." His mother asked "what on earth was wrong with him and he just stared at her, and paced the floor with both hands in his pockets." On other occasions he appeared in a daze, with a "glare in his eyes," and would not speak or respond to questions. In 1951, a few years after his discharge from the service, he "lost his mind and was pacing the floor saying something was after him." This incident occurred at the home of his aunt, Helen Calhoun. Disturbed by Robinson's conduct, Mrs. Calhoun called his mother about six o'clock in the morning, and she "went to see about him." Robinson tried to prevent Mrs. Calhoun from opening the door, saying "that someone was going to shoot him or someone was going to come in after him." His mother testified that, after gaining admittance, "I went to him and hugged him to ask him what was wrong and he went to pushing me back, telling me to get back, somebody was going to shoot him, somebody was going to shoot him." Upon being questioned as to Robinson's facial expression at the time, the mother stated that he "had that starey look and seemed to be just a little foamy at the mouth." A policeman was finally called. He put Robinson, his mother, and aunt in a cab which drove them to Hines Hospital. On the way Robinson tried to jump from the cab, and upon arrival at the hospital he was so violent that he had to be strapped in a wheel chair. He then was taken in an ambulance to the County Psychopathic Hospital, from which he was transferred to the Kankakee State Hospital. The medical records there recited:

> The reason for admission: The patient was admitted to this hospital on the 5th day of June, 1952, from the Hines Hospital. Patient began presenting symptoms of mental illness about a year ago at which time he came to his mother's house. He requested money and when it was refused, he suddenly kicked a hole in her bar. Was drinking and went to the Psychopathic Hospital. He imagined he heard voices, voices of men and women and he also saw things. He saw a little bit of everything. He saw animals, snakes and elephants and this lasted for about two days. He went to Hines. They sent him to the Psychopathic Hospital. The voices threatened him. He imagined someone was outside with a pistol aimed at him. He was very, very scared and he tried to call the police and his aunt then called the police. He thought he was going to be harmed. And he says this all seems very foolish to him now. Patient is friendly and tries to cooperate. He went through an acute toxic episode from which he has some insight. He had been drinking heavily. I am wondering possibly he isn't schizophrenic. I think he has recovered from this condition. I have seen the wife and she is in a pathetic state. I have no objection to giving him a try.

After his release from the state hospital Robinson's irrational episodes became more serious. His grandfather testified that while Robinson was working with him as a painter's assistant, "All at once, he would come down from the ladder and walk on out and never say where he is going and whatnot and he would be out two or three hours, and at times he would be in a daze and when he comes out, he comes back just as fresh. He just says he didn't do anything. I noticed that he wasn't at all himself." The grandfather also related that one night when Robinson was staying at his house Robinson and his wife had a "ruckus," which caused his wife to flee to the grandfather's bedroom. Robinson first tried to kick down the door. He then grabbed all of his wife's clothes from their room and threw them out in the yard, intending to set them on fire. Robinson got so unruly that the grandfather called the police to lock him up.

In 1953 Robinson, then separated from his wife, brought their 18-month-old son to Mrs. Calhoun's home and asked permission to stay there for a couple of days. She observed that he was highly nervous, prancing about and staring wildly. While she was at work the next day Robinson shot and killed his son and attempted suicide by shooting himself in the head. It appeared that after Robinson shot his son, he went to a nearby park and tried to take his life again by jumping into a lagoon. By his mother's description, he "was wandering around" the park, and walked up to a policeman and "asked him for a cigarette." It was stipulated that he went to the South Park Station on March 10, 1953, and said that he wanted to confess to a crime. When he removed his hat the police saw that he had shot himself in the head. They took him to the hospital for treatment of his wound.

> *In 1953, Robinson shot and killed his son and attempted suicide by shooting himself in the head.*

Robinson served almost four years in prison for killing his son, being released in September 1956. A few months thereafter he began to live with Flossie May Ward at her home. In the summer of 1957 or 1958 Robinson "jumped on" his mother's brother-in-law and "beat him up terrible." She went to the police station and swore out a warrant for his arrest. She described his abnormalities and told the officers that Robinson "seemed to have a disturbed mind." She asked the police "to pick him up so I can have him put away." Later she went back to see why they had not taken him into custody because of "the way he was fighting around in the streets, people were beating him up." She made another complaint a month or so before Robinson killed Flossie May Ward. However, no warrant was ever served on him.

The killing occurred about 10:30 p.m. at a small barbecue house where Flossie May Ward worked. At that time there were 10 customers in the restaurant, six of them sitting at the counter.

It appears from the record that Robinson entered the restaurant with a gun in his hand. As he approached the counter, Flossie May said, "Don't start nothing tonight." After staring at her for about a minute, he walked to the rear of the room and, with the use of his hand, leaped over the counter. He then rushed back toward the front of the restaurant, past two other employees working behind the counter, and fired once or twice at Flossie May. She jumped over the counter and ran out the front door with Robinson in pursuit. She was found dead on the sidewalk.[6] Robinson never spoke a word during the three-to-four-minute episode.

Subsequently Robinson went to the apartment of a friend, Mr. Moore, who summoned the police. When three officers, two in uniform, arrived, Robinson was standing in the hall approximately half way between the elevator and the apartment. Unaware of his identity, the officers walked past him and went to the door of the apartment. Mrs. Moore answered the door and told them that Robinson had left a short time earlier. As the officers turned around they saw Robinson still standing where they had first observed him. Robinson made no attempt to avoid being arrested. When asked his address he gave several evasive answers. He also denied knowing anything about the killing.[7]

Four defense witnesses expressed the opinion that Robinson was insane. In rebuttal the State introduced only a stipulation that Dr. William H. Haines, Director of the Behavior Clinic of the Criminal Court of Cook County would, if

> **It is contradictory to argue that a defendant may be incompetent, and yet knowingly or intelligently "waive" his right to have the court determine his capacity to stand trial.**

present, testify that in his opinion Robinson knew the nature of

---

[6] The Reverend Elmer Clemons was also shot and killed in the fracas. The indictment covering that offense was dismissed at the close of the trial in question.

[7] According to the testimony of an arresting officer the following exchange took place: "I asked him what his name was and he said, 'My name is Ted.' I said, 'What is your real name?' And he said, 'Theodore Robinson.' Then I asked him - I told him he was under arrest and he said, 'For what?' I said, 'Well, you are supposed to be wanted for killing two people on the south side.' I asked him did he know anything about it. He said, 'No, I don't know what you are talking about.' So then I asked him where he lived and he said, 'I don't live no place.' I said, 'What do you mean you don't live no place?' He said, 'That's what I said.' So then pretty soon I asked him again and he said, 'Sometimes I stay with my mother.' And I said, 'Where does she live?' He said, 'Some address on East 44th Street.' So then we took him on to the 27th District and while we were making the arrest slip, asked him again his address and he said he lived at 7320 South Parkway. That's about all he said. He didn't know anything about any killing or anything."

the charges against him and was able to cooperate with counsel when he examined him two or three months before trial. However, since the stipulation did not include a finding of sanity the prosecutor advised the court that "we should have Dr. Haines' testimony as to his opinion whether this man is sane or insane. It is possible that the man might be insane and know the nature of the charge or be able to cooperate with his counsel. I think it should be in evidence, your Honor, that Dr. Haines' opinion is that this defendant was sane when he was examined." However, the court told the prosecutor, "You have enough in the record now. I don't think you need Dr. Haines." In his summation defense counsel emphasized "Our defense is clear. It is as to the sanity of the defendant at the time of the crime and also as to the present time." The court, after closing argument by the defense, found Robinson guilty and sentenced him to prison for his natural life.

The State insists that Robinson deliberately waived the defense of his competence to stand trial by failing to demand a sanity hearing as provided by Illinois law. But it is contradictory to argue that a defendant may be incompetent, and yet knowingly or intelligently "waive" his right to have the court determine his capacity to stand trial. In any event, the record shows that counsel throughout the proceedings insisted that Robinson's present sanity

> While Robinson's demeanor at trial might be relevant to the ultimate decision as to his sanity, it cannot be relied upon to dispense with a hearing on that very issue.

was very much in issue. He made a point to elicit Mrs. Robinson's opinion of Robinson's "present sanity." And in his argument to the judge, he asserted that Robinson "should be found not guilty and presently insane on the basis of the testimony that we have heard." Moreover, the prosecutor himself suggested at trial that "we should have Dr. Haines' testimony as to his opinion whether this man is sane or insane." With this record we cannot say that Robinson waived the defense of incompetence to stand trial.[8]

We believe that the evidence introduced on Robinson's behalf entitled him to a hearing on this issue. The court's failure to

---

[8] Although defense counsel phrased his questions and argument in terms of Robinson's present insanity, we interpret his language as necessarily placing in issue the question of Robinson's mental competence to stand trial. Counsel was simply borrowing the terminology of the relevant Illinois statutes and decisions. The state law in effect at the time of Robinson's trial differentiated between lack of criminal responsibility and competence to stand trial, but used "insanity" to describe both concepts.

make such inquiry thus deprived Robinson of his constitutional right to a fair trial. Illinois jealously guards this right. Where the evidence raises a *"bona fide* doubt" as to a defendant's competence to stand trial, the judge on his own motion must impanel a jury and conduct a sanity hearing pursuant to [Illinois statute]. The Supreme Court of Illinois held that the evidence here was not sufficient to require a hearing in light of the mental alertness and understanding displayed in Robinson's "colloquies" with the trial judge. But this reasoning offers no justification for ignoring the uncontradicted testimony of Robinson's history of pronounced irrational behavior. While Robinson's demeanor at trial might be relevant to the ultimate decision as to his sanity, it cannot be relied upon to dispense with a hearing on that very issue. Likewise, the stipulation of Dr. Haines' testimony was some evidence of Robinson's ability to assist in his defense. But, as the state prosecutor seemingly admitted, on the facts presented to the trial court it could not properly have been deemed dispositive on the issue of Robinson's competence.[9]

Having determined that Robinson's constitutional rights were abridged by his failure to receive an adequate hearing on his competence to stand trial, we direct that the writ of *habeas corpus* must issue and Robinson be discharged, unless the State gives him a new trial within a reasonable time. It has been pressed upon us that it would be sufficient for the state court to hold a limited hearing as to Robinson's mental competence at the time he was tried in 1959. If he were found competent, the judgment against him would stand. But we have previously emphasized the difficulty of retrospectively determining an accused's competence to stand trial (*Dusky v. United States*). The jury would not be able to observe the subject of their inquiry, and expert witnesses would have to testify solely from information contained in the printed record. That Robinson's hearing would be held six years after the fact aggravates these difficulties. If the State elects to re-try Robinson, it will of course be open to him to raise the question of his competence to stand trial at that time and to request a special hearing thereon. In the event a sufficient doubt exists as to his present competence such a hearing must be held. If found

---

9 As defense counsel insisted in his closing argument: "In this case, which is a very serious case, the defendant has been able to cooperate with counsel with some reservations. However, I do not feel that this present lucidity bears on the issue of his sanity at the time of the crime and his sanity at the present time. I think the words sanity and insanity, the words are legal terms. I think that presently Mr. Theodore Robinson is in a lucid interval. I believe that from the witness stand you have heard testimony to indicate and prove that Mr. Theodore Robinson is presently insane."

competent to stand trial, Robinson would have the usual defenses available to an accused.

The case is remanded to the District Court for action consistent with this opinion.

It is so ordered.

Dissent: Mr. Justice Harlan, Whom Mr. Justice Black Joins, Dissenting

The facts now canvassed by this Court to support its constitutional holding were fully sifted by the Illinois Supreme Court. I cannot agree that the state court's unanimous appraisal was erroneous and still less that it was error of constitutional proportions.

The Court appears to hold that a defendant's present incompetence may become sufficiently manifest during a trial that it denies him due process for the trial court to fail to conduct a hearing on that question on its own initiative. I do not dissent from this very general proposition, and I agree also that such an error is not "waived" by failure to raise

> *The question, then, is not whether the facts before the trial judge suggested that Robinson's crime was an insane act but whether they suggested he was incompetent to stand trial. (Harlan, dissenting)*

it and that it may entitle the defendant to a new trial without further proof. However, I do not believe the facts known to the trial judge in this case suggested Robinson's incompetence at time of trial with anything like the force necessary to make out a violation of due process in the failure to pursue the question.

Before turning to the facts, it is pertinent to consider the quality of the incompetence they are supposed to indicate. In federal courts - and I assume no more is asked of state courts - the test of incompetence that warrants postponing the trial is reasonably well settled. In language this Court adopted on the one occasion it faced the issue, "the test must be whether the defendant has sufficient present ability to consult with his lawyer with a reasonable degree

> *Colloquies between Robinson and the trial judge undoubtedly permitted a reasonable inference that Robinson was quite cognizant of the proceedings and able to assist counsel in his defense. (Harlan, dissenting)*

of rational understanding - and whether he has a rational as well as factual understanding of the proceedings against him" (*Dusky*). In short, emphasis is on capacity to consult with counsel and to comprehend the proceedings, and lower courts have recognized that this is by no means the same test as those which determine criminal responsibility at the time of the crime.

The question, then, is not whether the facts before the trial judge suggested that Robinson's crime was an insane act but whether they suggested he was incompetent to stand trial. The Court's affirmative answer seemingly rests on two kinds of evidence, principally adduced by Robinson to prove an insanity defense after the State rested its main case. First, there was evidence of a number of episodes of severe irrationality in Robinson's past. The second class of data pertinent to the Court's theory, remarks by witnesses and counsel that Robinson was "presently insane," deserves little comment. I think it apparent that these statements were addressed to Robinson's responsibility for the killing, that is, his ability to do insane acts, and not to his general competency to stand trial.

Whatever mild doubts this evidence may stir are surely allayed by positive indications of Robinson's competence at the trial. Foremost is his own behavior in the courtroom. The record reveals colloquies between Robinson and the trial judge which undoubtedly permitted a reasonable inference that Robinson was quite cognizant of the proceedings and able to assist counsel in his defense. Turning from lay impressions to those of an expert, it was stipulated at trial that a Dr. Haines, Director of the Behavior Clinic of the

> *Robinson's own lawyers, the two men who apparently had the closest contact with the defendant during the proceedings, never suggested he was incompetent to stand trial and never moved to have him examined on incompetency grounds during trial. (Harlan, dissenting)*

Criminal Court of Cook County, had examined Robinson several months earlier and, if called, would testify that Robinson "knows the nature of the charge and is able to cooperate with his counsel." The conclusive factor is that Robinson's own lawyers, the two men who apparently had the closest contact with the defendant during the proceedings, never suggested he was incompetent to stand trial and never moved to have him examined on incompetency grounds during trial; indeed, counsel's remarks to the jury seem best read as an affirmation of Robinson's present "lucidity" which would be highly peculiar if Robinson had been unable to assist properly in his defense.

Thus, I cannot agree with the Court that the requirements of due process were violated by the failure of the trial judge, who had opportunities for personal observation of the defendant that we do not possess, to halt the trial and hold a competency hearing on his own motion.

In my view, the Court of Appeals should be reversed and the District Court's dismissal of the petition reinstated.

Drope v. Missouri

420 U.S. 302 (1975)

Facts

In 1969, James Edward Drope and two others were indicted for the rape of Drope's wife. Drope filed a motion for a continuance so he might be examined and receive psychiatric care, if needed. Attached to the motion was a report by a psychiatrist who had previously examined Drope at his counsel's request and had suggested such treatment. The motion for a continuance was denied, and the case proceeded to trial. Drope's wife testified at trial, repeating and confirming information contained in the psychiatric report regarding "strange behavior" exhibited by Drope. She also testified that her husband had tried to kill her the Sunday prior to trial. On the morning of the second day of trial, Drope shot himself in the stomach in an alleged suicide attempt. Because he was hospitalized and therefore unable to be present for the remainder of the trial, defense counsel moved for a mistrial. The motion was denied on the ground that Drope's absence was voluntary, having been brought about by his own actions. The trial continued, and the jury returned a verdict of guilty. Drope received a sentence of life imprisonment.

Procedural History

Drope filed a motion for a new trial, alleging the trial court had erred in proceeding with the trial without sufficient evidence that Drope's absence from trial was voluntary. The motion was denied. Thereafter, Drope filed a motion to vacate the judgment of conviction and sentence, alleging his constitutional rights had been violated by the failure to order a psychiatric examination prior to trial and by conducting the trial to conclusion in his absence. The motion to vacate was denied, and the Missouri Court of Appeals affirmed. The U.S. Supreme Court granted *certiorari*[1] and reversed.

Issue

What is the threshold for ordering a competency evaluation?

---

[1] *certiorari.* A means of gaining appellate review.

Holding

Due process requires that where there is sufficient doubt as to a defendant's competence to stand trial, further inquiry is required.

Analysis

It has long been accepted that a person whose mental condition is such that he lacks the capacity to understand the nature and purpose of the proceedings against him, to consult with counsel, and to assist in preparing his defense may not be subjected to a trial. The failure to observe procedures adequate to protect a defendant's right not to be tried or convicted while incompetent to stand trial deprives him of his due process rights to a fair trial.

In the opinion of the Supreme Court, the Missouri trial court failed to give proper weight to information suggesting Drope's incompetence to stand trial and thereby failed to initiate an inquiry. This failure constituted a violation of due process of law. The Court stated that when considered in conjunction with information available prior to trial (e.g., the psychiatric report) and information provided during trial (e.g., the testimony of Drope's wife), information concerning Drope's suicide attempt created a "sufficient doubt" of his competence to stand trial so as to require further inquiry. The suicide attempt reportedly suggested "a rather substantial degree of mental instability contemporaneous with the trial," and his absence from court prevented the trial judge and defense counsel from being able to observe him in the context of the trial in order to "gauge from his demeanor whether he was able to cooperate with his attorney and to understand the nature and object of the proceedings against him."

In sum, the Court noted that evidence of a defendant's irrational behavior, his demeanor at trial, and any prior medical opinion on competence to stand trial are all relevant in determining whether further inquiry is required. Even one of these factors standing alone may, in some circumstances, be sufficient; there are no fixed or immutable signs that invariably indicate the need for further inquiry. Additionally, even when a defendant is competent at the commencement of trial, the trial court must always be alert to circumstances suggesting a change that would render the accused unable to meet the standards of competence to stand trial.

Edited Excerpts[2]

James Edward Drope v. State of Missouri

Supreme Court of the United States

420 U.S. 302

February 19, 1975

Certiorari to the Court of Appeals of Missouri for the
St. Louis District

Mr. Chief Justice Burger
Delivered the Opinion of the Court

We granted *certiorari*[3] in this case to consider petitioner's
claims that he was deprived of due process of law by the failure of
the trial court to order a psychiatric examination with respect to
his competence to stand trial and by the conduct in his absence of
a portion of his trial on an indictment charging a capital offense.

In February 1969 an indictment was returned in the Circuit
Court of St. Louis, Missouri, charging petitioner and two others
with the forcible rape of petitioner's wife. Following severance of
petitioner's case from
those of the other defendants and a continuance,
on May 27 his counsel
filed a motion for a con-
tinuance until Septem-

> **Petitioner's attorney moved for a
> mistrial in view of the fact that the
> defendant shot himself. The trial
> judge denied the motion.**

ber, in order that petitioner might be examined and receive psychiatric treatment. Treatment had been suggested by a psychiatrist who had examined petitioner at his counsel's request and
whose report was attached to the motion.[4] On the same date re-

---

[2] Readers are advised to quote only from the original published cases. See pages
vii-viii.

[3] *certiorari.* A means of gaining appellate review.

[4] The report describes petitioner as "markedly agitated and upset," noting that he
"appeared to be cooperative in this examination, but he had difficulty in participating well." The report continues: "The patient had a difficult time relating. He
was markedly circumstantial and irrelevant in his speech. There was no sign as
to the presence of any delusions, illusions, hallucinations, obsessions, ideas of
reference, compulsions or phobias at this time."

The report then recounts the details of a conversation between the psychiatrist and petitioner's wife. The latter admitted that she had left petitioner on a
number of occasions because of his sexual perversions and described the

spondent, through the Assistant Circuit Attorney, filed a document stating that the State did not oppose the motion for a psychiatric examination. Apparently no action was taken on the motion, and petitioner's case was continued until June 23, at which time his counsel objected to proceeding with the trial on the ground that he had understood the case would be continued until September and consequently was not prepared. He objected further "for the reason that the defendant is not a person of sound mind and should have a further psychiatric examination before the case should be forced to trial." The trial judge noted that the motion for a continuance was not in proper form and that, although petitioner's counsel had agreed to file another, he had failed to do so, and he overruled his objections and directed that the case proceed to trial.

On June 24 a jury was impaneled, and the prosecution called petitioner's wife as its first witness. She testified that petitioner participated with four of his acquaintances in forcibly raping her and subjecting her to other bizarre abuse and indignities, but that she had resumed living with him after the incident on the advice of petitioner's psychiatrist and so that their children would be taken care of. On cross-examination, she testified that she had told petitioner's attorney of her belief that her husband was sick and needed psychiatric care and that for these reasons she had signed a statement disavowing a desire to prosecute. She related that on several occasions when petitioner did not "get his way or was worried about something," he would roll down the stairs. She could explain such behavior only by relating "what they told him many times at City Hospital, that is something he does upon himself." However, she also stated that she was not convinced petitioner was sick after talking to his psychiatrist, and that she had changed her mind about not wanting to prosecute petitioner because, as she testified, he had "tried to choke me, tried to kill me" on the Sunday evening prior to trial.

The prosecution called three more witnesses, but did not conclude its case, before adjournment on June 24. The following morning, petitioner did not appear. When the trial judge directed

---

"strange behavior" of petitioner, including falling down flights of stairs, as an attempt to gain sympathy from her. In a section entitled "Impression," the report states that petitioner had "always led a marginal existence," that he had a "history of anti-social conduct," but that there were no "strong signs of psychosis at this time." It concludes that petitioner "certainly needs the aid of a psychiatrist," and that he "is a very neurotic individual who is also depressed and perhaps he is depressed for most of the time," and it offers as diagnoses: "(1) Sociopathic personality disorder, sexual perversion. (2) Borderline mental deficiency. (3) Chronic Anxiety reaction with depression."

counsel to proceed, petitioner's attorney moved for a mistrial "in view of the fact that the defendant, I am informed, shot himself this morning." The trial judge denied the motion, stating that he had already decided the matter would proceed for trial, and when petitioner's counsel complained of the difficulty of proceeding without a client, the trial judge replied that the difficulty was brought about by petitioner, who was on bond and had a responsibility to be present. The jury returned a verdict of guilty, and on July 21, 1969, petitioner, who had been in the hospital for three weeks recovering from a bullet wound in the abdomen, appeared, and the trial court fixed the penalty at life imprisonment.

Petitioner filed a motion for a new trial, the burden of which was that the trial court had erred in proceeding with the trial when no evidence had been produced that his absence from the trial was voluntary. A hearing was held before the judge who had presided at trial. Petitioner testified that on June 25 he had gone to his brother's house and that he remembered nothing concerning the shooting except that he felt a burn-

> **The mentally incompetent defendant, though physically present in the courtroom, is in reality afforded no opportunity to defend himself.**

ing pain in his stomach and later woke up in the hospital. He testified he did not remember talking to anyone at the hospital. The State presented evidence that upon admission to the hospital petitioner stated that he had shot himself because of "some problem with the law," and that he had told a policeman he had shot himself because "he was supposed to go to court for rape, and he didn't do it; he rather be dead than to go to trial for something he didn't do." The trial judge denied the motion. Stating that on the morning of petitioner's failure to appear he had received information on the telephone which was checked with the hospital, the judge concluded that petitioner had the burden of showing that his absence was not voluntary and found on the basis of the evidence that his absence "was due to his own voluntary act in shooting himself; done for the very purpose of avoiding trial." We granted *certiorari*, and we now reverse.

It has long been accepted that a person whose mental condition is such that he lacks the capacity to understand the nature and object of the proceedings against him, to consult with counsel, and to assist in preparing his defense may not be subjected to a trial. Thus, Blackstone[5] wrote that one who became "mad" after the commission of an offense should not be arraigned for it "be-

---

[5] Blackstone. Famous legal scholar.

cause he is not able to plead to it with that advice and caution that he ought." Similarly, if he became "mad" after pleading, he should not be tried, "for how can he make his defense?" Some have viewed the common-law prohibition "as a by-product of the ban against trials *in absentia*; the mentally incompetent defendant, though physically present in the courtroom, is in reality afforded no opportunity to defend himself." For our purposes, it suffices to note that the prohibition is fundamental to an adversary system of justice. Accordingly, as to federal cases, we have approved a test of incompetence which seeks to ascertain whether a criminal defendant "has sufficient present ability to consult with his lawyer with a reasonable degree of rational understanding - and whether he has a rational as well as factual understanding of the proceedings against him" (*Dusky*).

As was true of Illinois in *Pate*, Missouri's statutory scheme "jealously guards" a defendant's right to a fair trial: "No person who as a result of mental disease or defect lacks capacity to understand the proceedings against him or to assist in his own defense shall be tried, convicted or sentenced for the commission of an offense so long as the incapacity endures." [The statute] provides that a judge or magistrate shall, "upon his own motion or upon motion filed by the state or by or on behalf of the accused," order a psychiatric examination whenever he "has reasonable cause to believe that the accused has a mental disease or defect excluding fitness to proceed." Such a procedure is, on its face, constitutionally adequate to protect a defendant's right not to be tried while legally incompetent. Our task is to determine whether the proceedings in this case were consistent with petitioner's right to a fair trial.

In the present case there is no dispute as to the evidence possibly relevant to petitioner's mental condition that was before the trial court prior to trial and thereafter. Rather, the dispute concerns the inferences that were to be drawn from the undisputed evidence and whether, in light of what was then known, the failure to make further inquiry into petitioner's competence to stand trial denied him a fair trial. In such circumstances we believe it is "incumbent upon us to analyze the facts in

> *Petitioner's suicide attempt created a sufficient doubt of his competence to stand trial to require further inquiry on the question.*

order that the appropriate enforcement of the federal right may be assured."

The sentencing judge and the Missouri Court of Appeals concluded that the psychiatric evaluation of petitioner attached to his pretrial motion for a continuance did not contain sufficient indicia of incompetence to stand trial to require further inquiry. Both courts mentioned aspects of the report suggesting competence, such as the impressions that petitioner did not have "any delusions, illusions, hallucinations," was "well oriented in all spheres," and "was able, without trouble, to answer questions testing judgement," but neither court mentioned the contrary data. The report also showed that petitioner, although cooperative in the examination, "had difficulty in participating well," "had a difficult time relating," and that he "was markedly circumstantial and irrelevant in his speech." In addition, neither court felt that petitioner's episodic irrational acts described in the report or the psychiatrist's diagnoses of "borderline mental deficiency" and "chronic anxiety reaction with depression" created a sufficient doubt of competence to require further inquiry.

It does not appear that the examining psychiatrist was asked to address himself to medical facts bearing specifically on the issue of petitioner's competence to stand trial, as distinguished from his mental and emotional condition generally. Thus, it is not surprising that before this Court the dispute centers on the inferences that could or should properly have been drawn from the report. Even where the issue is in focus we have recognized "the uncertainty of diagnosis in this field and the tentativeness of professional judgment" (*Greenwood v. United States*). Here the inquiry is rendered more difficult by the fact that a defendant's mental condition may be relevant to more than one legal issue, each governed by distinct rules reflecting quite different policies. See *Jackson v. Indiana*.

Like the report itself, the motion for a continuance did not clearly suggest that petitioner's competence to stand trial was the question sought to be resolved. While we have expressed doubt that the right to further inquiry upon the question can be waived, see *Pate*, it is nevertheless true that judges must depend to some extent on counsel to bring issues into focus. Petitioner's somewhat inartfully drawn motion for a continuance probably fell short of appropriate assistance to the trial court in that regard. However, we are constrained to disagree with the sentencing judge that counsel's pretrial contention that "the defendant is not a person of sound mind and should have a further psychiatric examination before the case should be forced to trial," did not raise the issue of petitioner's competence to stand trial. This statement also may have tended to blur the aspect of petitioner's mental condition which would bear on his criminal responsibility and that which would bear on his competence to stand trial. However, at that stage, and with the obvious advantages of hindsight, it seems to us that it would have been, at the very least, the better practice to order an immediate examination under [Missouri statute]. It is unnecessary for us to decide whether such examination was constitutionally required on the basis of what was then known to the trial court since in our view the question was settled by later events.

Turning to the situation at petitioner's trial, the state courts viewed the evidence as failing to show that during trial petitioner had acted in a manner that would cause the trial court to doubt his competence. The testimony of petitioner's wife, some of which repeated and confirmed in-

> **The fact that Mr. Drope shot himself to avoid trial suggests very strongly an awareness of what was going on. (Sentencing judge)**

formation contained in the psychiatric evaluation attached to petitioner's motion for a continuance, was given little weight. Finally, the sentencing judge, relying on his finding on petitioner's motion for a new trial and although stating "that it does not take a psychiatrist to know that such a man has a problem and indicates poor judgment," concluded that the "fact that Mr. Drope shot himself to avoid trial suggests very strongly an awareness of what was going on." The Missouri Court of Appeals, accepting *arguendo*[6] petitioner's contention that his was "a *bona fide* attempt at suicide," refused to conclude "that as a matter of law an attempt at suicide creates a reasonable doubt as to the movant's competency to stand trial."

Notwithstanding the difficulty of making evaluations of the kind required in these circumstances, we conclude that the record reveals a failure to give proper weight to the information suggesting incompetence which came to light during trial. This is particularly so when viewed in the context of the events surrounding petitioner's suicide attempt and against the background of the pretrial showing. Although a defendant's demeanor during trial may be such as to obviate "the need for extensive reliance on psychiatric prediction concerning his capabilities," we concluded in *Pate* that "this reasoning offers no justification for ignoring the uncontradicted testimony of a history of pronounced irrational behavior." We do not mean to suggest that the indicia of such behavior in this case approximated those in *Pate*, but we believe the Missouri courts failed to consider and give proper weight to the record evidence. Too little weight was given to the testimony of petitioner's wife that on the Sunday prior to trial he tried to choke her to death. For a man whose fate depended in large measure on

---

[6] *arguendo*. For the sake of argument.

the indulgence of his wife, who had hesitated about pressing the prosecution, this hardly could be regarded as rational conduct. Moreover, in considering the indicia of petitioner's incompetence separately, the state courts gave insufficient attention to the aggregate of those indicia in applying the objective standard of [Missouri statute]. We need not address the Court of Appeals' conclusion that an attempt to commit suicide does not create a reasonable doubt of competence to stand trial as a matter of law. As was true of the psychiatric evaluation, petitioner's attempt to commit suicide "did not stand alone." We conclude that when considered together with the information available prior to trial and the testimony of petitioner's wife at trial, the information concerning petitioner's suicide attempt created a sufficient doubt of his competence to stand trial to require further inquiry on the question.

The import of our decision in *Pate* is that evidence of a defendant's irrational behavior, his demeanor at trial, and any prior medical opinion on competence to stand trial are all relevant in determining whether further inquiry is required, but that even one of these factors standing alone may, in some circumstances, be sufficient. There are, of course, no fixed or immutable signs which invariably indicate the need for further

> **There are, of course, no fixed or immutable signs which invariably indicate the need for further inquiry to determine fitness to proceed.**

inquiry to determine fitness to proceed; the question is often a difficult one in which a wide range of manifestations and subtle nuances are implicated. That they are difficult to evaluate is suggested by the varying opinions trained psychiatrists can entertain on the same facts.

Here, the evidence of irrational behavior prior to trial was weaker than in *Pate*, but there was no opinion evidence as to petitioner's competence to stand trial. Moreover, Robinson was present throughout his trial; [here] petitioner was absent for a crucial portion of his trial. Petitioner's absence bears on the analysis in two ways: first, it was due to an act which suggests a rather substantial degree of mental instability contemporaneous with the trial;[7] as a result of petitioner's absence the trial judge and

---

[7] We assume, as did the Missouri Court of Appeals, that petitioner's was a "*bona fide*" suicide attempt, rather than, as [the government] contends, malingering. In that regard, the hearsay information in the possession of the trial judge when he denied the motion for a mistrial suggested an intent on the part of petitioner to kill himself, and a self-inflicted wound near vital organs does not suggest malingering. Of course we also recognize that "the empirical relation-

defense counsel were no longer able to observe him in the context of the trial and to gauge from his demeanor whether he was able to cooperate with his attorney and to understand the nature and object of the proceedings against him.

Even when a defendant is competent at the commencement of his trial, a trial court must always be alert to circumstances suggesting a change that would render the accused unable to meet the standards of competence to stand trial. Whatever the relationship between mental illness and incompetence to stand trial, in this case the bearing of the former on the latter was sufficiently likely that, in light of the evidence of petitioner's behavior including his suicide attempt, and there being no opportunity without his presence to evaluate that bearing in fact, the correct course was to suspend the trial until such an evaluation could be made. That this might have aborted the trial is a hard reality, but we cannot fail to note that such a result might have been avoided by prompt psychiatric examination before trial, when it was sought by petitioner.

The Missouri Court of Appeals concluded that, had further inquiry into petitioner's competence to stand trial been constitutionally mandated in this case, it would have been permissible to defer it until the trial had been completed. Such a procedure may have advantages, at least where the defendant is present at the trial and the appropriate inquiry is implemented with dispatch. However, because of petitioner's absence during a critical stage of his trial, neither the judge nor counsel was able to observe him, and the hearing on his motion for a new trial, held approximately three months after the trial, was not informed by an inquiry into either his competence to stand trial or his capacity effectively to waive his right to be present. The question remains whether petitioner's due process rights would be adequately protected by remanding the case now for a psychiatric examination aimed at establishing whether petitioner was in fact competent to stand trial in 1969. Given the inherent difficulties of such a *nunc*

> *Even when a defendant is competent at the commencement of his trial, a trial court must always be alert to circumstances suggesting a change that would render the accused unable to meet the standards of competence to stand trial.*

---

ship between mental illness and suicide" or suicide attempts is uncertain and that a suicide attempt need not always signal "an inability to perceive reality accurately, to reason logically and to make plans and carry them out in an organized fashion."

pro tunc[8] determination under the most favorable circumstances, we cannot conclude that such a procedure would be adequate here. The State is free to re-try petitioner, assuming, of course, that at the time of such trial he is competent to be tried.

The judgment is reversed, and the cause is remanded for proceedings not inconsistent with this opinion.

---

[8] *nunc pro tunc* determination. Supplementing a prior determination.

Seidner v. United States

260 F.2d 732 (D.C. Cir., 1958)

Facts

Albert Seidner was tried for attempted extortion. Midway through the government's case, Seidner announced his desire to plead guilty to the lesser offense of sending a threatening letter through the mail. He addressed the court for approximately 30 minutes to explain why he wished to change his plea. Because his statements to the court indicated to the prosecutor that Seidner might be suffering delusions of persecution, the prosecutor moved for a mental health examination. Seidner's counsel opposed the motion, and the trial judge, after hearing argument, denied the motion without prejudice.[1] Before sentencing, Seidner's counsel assured the judge he had personally checked into the truth of the statements Seidner made in changing his plea, and had found some of them to be true. So satisfied, the judge pronounced sentence. Upon receiving a letter from Seidner indicating he was incarcerated in a Bureau of Prisons mental institution, and after examining the records, the Court of Appeals for the District of Columbia Circuit appointed a member of the bar as *amicus curiae*[2] to investigate and file a memorandum. The memorandum raised for the first time a question as to whether the appellant had been competent at the time of the trial. Seidner rejected the idea he may have been incompetent.

Issue

Can the issue of a defendant's competency to stand trial be raised, against the defendant's wishes, after defendant has been convicted and sentenced?

Holding

Yes. The record before the Court of Appeals warranted judicial inquiry concerning Seidner's competency when he changed

---

[1] *without prejudice.* Indicates the issue can be raised again.
[2] *amicus curiae.* "Friend of the court"; interested person or group not party to the case.

his plea and was sentenced. If Seidner was incompetent when he pleaded guilty, the sentence must be vacated.

Analysis

If Seidner was indeed mentally incompetent, the court could not rely upon his decision regarding whether the competency issue was to be raised prior to trial. Instead, the trial court could have appointed counsel to represent the appellant's interests, or if he persisted in refusing counsel, the court could have appointed an *amicus curiae* to present the case independently. The objective must be to achieve fundamental fairness bearing in mind that rigid rules of procedure, or evidence, or order of proof, will not always best serve the interests of substantial justice when applied to a post-conviction proceeding.

Edited Excerpts[3]

Albert Seidner, Appellant v. United States of America

United States Court of Appeals, District of Columbia Circuit

260 F.2d 732

November 17, 1958

Before Prettyman, Bazelon, and Burger, Circuit Judges

per curiam[4]

Upon receiving a letter from appellant which indicated he was incarcerated in a mental institution run by the Bureau of Prisons and after examining the records, this court appointed a member of the bar as *amicus curiae* to file a memorandum. The memorandum raised for the first time a question as to whether appellant had been mentally competent at the time of his trial.

In response to a show cause order which this court issued after considering the *amicus* memorandum, the Director of Prisons stated that he had examined the report made by the Lewisburg Prison Board of Examiners of its psychiatric examination of ap-

---

[3] Readers are advised to quote only from the original published cases. See pages vii-viii.

[4] *per curiam*. By the court, no single opinion writer identified.

pellant, an examination made six and one-half months after sentence on a guilty plea. The Director found therein no probable cause to believe that appellant was mentally incompetent at the time of his plea. However, the present state of the record suggests it is possible that there is some question concerning appellant's competency to stand trial.

If appellant was incompetent when he pleaded guilty, the sentence must be vacated. Appellant, however, rejects the idea he may have been incompetent. Despite his protests, we hold that the issue of competency is cognizable. Accordingly we remand in order that the District Court may now determine whether the issue of competency requires that the sentence be vacated, conviction at new trial reversed on other grounds, or whether on the other hand a determination of appellant's competency can be made *nunc pro tunc*.[5]

> **If appellant was incompetent when he pleaded guilty, the sentence must be vacated.**

Bazelon, Concurring

The question of appellant's mental condition at the time of the trial first came to our notice when appellant requested authority to be brought to Washington, DC, from the Medical Center for Federal Prisoners at Springfield, Missouri, for the purpose of arguing his appeal. Upon inquiry as to why appellant was confined at the Medical Center, we were advised he was a "certified psychotic." We thereupon appointed a member of the bar as *amicus curiae* to investigate and file a memorandum.

The memorandum and other records show the following: Appellant went to trial on an indictment for attempted extortion. Midway through the government's case, appellant announced his desire to plead guilty to a lesser offense of sending a threatening letter through the mails. Appellant addressed the court for some thirty minutes to explain why he wished to change his plea. Apparently because appellant's statements to the court indicated to the prosecutor that appellant might be suffering delusions of persecution,

> **Unless the court is satisfied by a clear preponderance of all the evidence that appellant was competent when tried, the judgment of conviction be set aside. (Bazelon, concurring)**

---

[5] *nunc pro tunc* determination. Supplementing a prior determination.

the prosecutor moved for a mental examination of appellant. Appellant's counsel opposed the Government's motion. Before sentence was pronounced, appellant's counsel assured the judge that he had personally checked into the truth of appellant's statements in changing his plea, and that counsel found some of them to be true. So satisfied, the judge sentenced appellant to serve from one to three years, and appellant was sent to the penitentiary at Lewisburg, Pennsylvania.

Appellant has served notice that he will oppose any determination that he was incompetent to stand trial. He cannot therefore be expected to consult with any counsel who may be appointed to assist him at the hearing. Moreover, since the Prison Bureau has classified appellant as a "certified psychotic" in the recent past, his participation in any proceeding now is a delicate matter requiring great caution. These matters make clear that the hearing cannot be an adversary one. I think they require that (1) the Government proceed first, (2) the court take the initiative in ordering the presentation of any evidence which promises to shed light on the issue, and (3) unless the court is satisfied by a clear preponderance of all the evidence that appellant was competent when tried, the judgment of conviction be set aside.

Implications for Examiners

Competency is determined by a defendant's present abilities. In *Kenner*, the court relied on stale mental health evaluations. Although two motions for a competency evaluation were made in 1959, the trial court in *Kenner* relied on information about the defendant's mental state in 1952 and 1953. Clinicians recognize that debilitating periods of mental illness can be intermittent and that an individual's capabilities may be difficult to predict even in the short term. *Kenner* highlights the importance of informing courts that changes in mental state are commonly observed. Psychologists and psychiatrists can often assist a court by providing information about the nature of specific symptoms or the course of a particular disorder. Similarly, experts should offer prognostic statements regarding the stability of an individual's current condition, as well as a discussion of variables that may maintain or disrupt a defendant's mental state.

Some decisions at Robinson's first trial (in *Pate*) stemmed from confusing statutory language. At the time of this case, Illinois statutes used the term "sanity" to connote both competency and mental state at the time of the offense. Experts must understand the meaning of the language in the jurisdictions in which they perform evaluations. In many courts, questions about competency may be a low-frequency occurrence. As such, legal professionals may not be familiar with the relevant issues, much less the language necessary to effectively communicate their concerns. Such confusion is evident when courts ask about a person's "competency at the time of the offense." It is incumbent on the expert to clarify, for themselves and sometimes for the court, the relevant mental health issues in a given case.

The Supreme Court decision in *Drope* indicates courts generally require the expertise of psychologists and psychiatrists to interpret unusual behavior. In Drope's case, one could question whether he had a major mental illness. Based on the facts in the case, it certainly appears plausible that he had a personality disorder and not a major mental disorder. Clearly, his judgment was terribly flawed. (His wife had chosen not to testify against him, until he assaulted her shortly before the trial.) The trial court judge appeared to make a common-sense judgment about Drope's actions and viewed them as voluntary misbehavior. The Supreme Court ruled that the trial court did not have sufficient basis to make that interpretation. Instead, the Supreme Court ruled that Drope's unusual behaviors were sufficient to trigger an evaluation. Expert evaluation may have provided the trial court with the information necessary to confirm the common-sense conclusion that Drope was simply misbehaving, or it may have revealed a major mental illness that contributed to or caused the defendant's bizarre behavior. Regardless of the findings of evaluations, courts profit when experts explain factors which influence thought, emotion, and behavior. In *Drope*, the court would have benefited from an explanation of the likely cause of this defendant's poor judgment.

The decisions in both *Pate* and *Drope* establish a low threshold for referring defendants for mental health evaluation. Any *bona fide* doubt is sufficient to trigger a competency evaluation. In practice, this low standard affects the base rates of competency and incompetency for defendants evaluated by psychologists and psychiatrists. As a result, many competent defendants will be referred for competency evaluations. Whereas a naive observer might think a fair expert would find defendants competent and incompetent in equal numbers, clinicians should recognize that the low threshold for referrals leads to a different circumstance: Most defendants are competent.

Seidner is also related to the threshold for referral for an evaluation. In this case, a conviction was overturned when the appellate court determined, after the fact, that the defendant had been incompetent at the time of the conviction. A lower threshold for an evaluation may have prevented the situation faced by the appellate court in *Seidner*. This 1958 decision predated both *Pate* and *Drope*. It is reasonable to conclude that the guidelines set forth in those cases decrease the likelihood of erroneous convictions of incompetent defendants. Nevertheless, experts may occasionally face questions regarding a defendant's competency at a previous point in time, thus necessitating a retrospective evaluation of the individual's abilities.

Section 3

Constitutional And Judicial Considerations

Introduction to Section 3

Cases

Implications for Examiners

Introduction to Section 3

This section concerns the potential for paradigm clashes between mental health experts and the courts. *McDonald v. United States* (1962) is a case primarily concerned with criminal responsibility. We include it because it speaks to the issue of tension between what courts and clinicians consider mental disorder to be, an issue clearly relevant to determinations of competency. According to the *McDonald* decision in the Court of Appeals for the District of Columbia Circuit, "What mental health professionals may consider a mental disease or defect for clinical purposes may or may not be the same as mental disease or defect for the jury's purposes in determining criminal responsibility."

In *Medina v. California* (1992), the U.S. Supreme Court held that a state may require a defendant claiming incompetence to stand trial to bear the burden of proving incompetence by a preponderance of the evidence. The presumption of competence does not violate due process. The U.S. Supreme Court ruled in *Cooper v. Oklahoma* (1996) that preponderance of evidence was the appropriate standard for competency determinations. Oklahoma had required Cooper to prove he was competent by clear and convincing evidence. Difficulty in ascertaining whether a defendant is incompetent or malingering may make it appropriate to place the burden of proof on a defendant, but it does not justify the additional burden of an especially high standard of proof.

In *Godinez v. Moran* (1993), the U.S. Supreme Court held that *Dusky* provides a single standard of competence, whether it is competence to stand trial or to plead guilty. Although mental health experts might find it useful to distinguish among various abilities and task demands related to resolving legal charges, the only standard for competency is a rational and factual appreciation of one's circumstances and an ability to properly assist one's attorney. The U.S. Supreme Court held in *North Carolina v. Alford* (1970) that the standard for determining the validity of a guilty plea is whether the plea represents a voluntary and intelligent choice among the alternative courses of action available to the defendant. Alford complained that his guilty plea for murder was coerced because going to trial entailed a high risk of receiving the death penalty. The Supreme Court said this did not render the plea invalid; it was the product of a free and rational choice.

In *United States v. Greer* (1998), the Court of Appeals for the Fifth Circuit held that the right to a competency evaluation does not include the right to *create* a doubt about competency. Greer appealed an increase in his sentence based on the trial judge's conclusion that by feigning mental disorder, he had obstructed justice. Greer's appeal was denied.

McDonald v. United States

312 F.2d 847 (D.C. Cir., 1962)

Facts

Ernest McDonald was convicted of manslaughter and sentenced to from 5 to 15 years imprisonment. Evidence presented at trial included testimony that defendant had a "mental defect" (based on an IQ of 68 and other evidence of "mental abnormality").

Issue

Was there sufficient evidence of mental disease or defect to require an instruction on criminal responsibility?

Holding

If there is some evidence supporting a claim of mental disability, the defendant is entitled to have that issue submitted to the jury. Evidence of mental disease or defect raises the issue of mental disability.

Analysis

What mental health professionals may consider a mental disease or defect for clinical purposes may or may not be the same as mental disease or defect for the jury's purposes in determining criminal responsibility. The jury should be instructed that "mental disease" or "mental defect" includes "any abnormal condition of the mind substantially affecting mental or emotional processes and substantially impairing behavior controls." Furthermore, the trier of fact is the ultimate decision maker as to whether a mental disease or defect exists.

Edited Excerpts[1]

Ernest McDonald, Appellant, v. United States of America,
Appellee

United States Court of Appeals District of Columbia Circuit

312 F.2d 847

October 8, 1962

Before Wilbur K. Miller, Chief Judge, and Edgerton,
Bazelon, Fahy, Washington, Danaher, Bastian,
Burger and Wright, Circuit Judges, sitting *en banc*[2]

per curiam[3]

Appellant was convicted of manslaughter and sentenced to
from five to fifteen years imprisonment. He had been charged
with second degree murder for aiding and abetting his employer
in the shooting of one Jenkins during an altercation.

[The court] twice enumerated the alternative verdicts available to the jury. But both times it failed to include "not guilty because of insanity." The government urges that the evidence was
insufficient to require an instruction on responsibility, hence any
defects in the instruction are immaterial. We do not agree that
the instruction was unnecessary.

In this case a psychiatrist and a psychologist testified that the
defendant had a "mental defect," principally because his IQ rating shown by various tests was below the "average" intelligence
range of 90 to 110. His overall IQ was 68. Neither witness was
able to say whether ap-
pellant's mental defect
stemmed from organic in-
jury or from some other
cause. But the psychiatrist

> **Evidence of a 68 IQ rating, stand-
> ing alone and without more, is not
> evidence of a "mental defect."**

testified that some organic pathology can only be established by
autopsy and that McDonald's defect probably prevented him from
progressing beyond the sixth grade.

---

[1] Readers are advised to quote only from the original published cases. See pages
vii-viii.

[2] *en banc*. All the judges of an appellate court considering an opinion together.

[3] *per curiam*. By the court, no single opinion writer identified.

The witnesses also explained generally how mental defect affects behavior. The psychologist testified that a person suffering from a mental defect would have less ability than normal persons to distinguish between right and wrong in complex situations; would tend to act impulsively under stress; and would readily become dependent upon and be strongly influenced by someone who befriended him. The witness testified further that McDonald had a mental defect, which she defined as "a state of mental development which does not reach the level of average intelligence," and that "if McDonald had a person on whom he was dependent and if that person should produce a gun and threaten another McDonald would not be as able as the average adult to assess and evaluate the situation and the consequences of whatever action he might take." The psychiatrist stated that McDonald would lack the ability of normal persons to foresee the consequences of his acts.

Evidence of a 68 IQ rating, standing alone and without more, is not evidence of a "mental defect." Our purpose now is to make it very clear that neither the court nor the jury is bound by *ad hoc* definitions or conclusions as to what experts state is a disease or defect. What psychiatrists may consider a "mental disease or defect" for clinical purposes, where their concern is treatment, may or may not be the same as mental disease or defect for the jury's purpose in determining criminal responsibility. Consequently, for that purpose the jury should be told that a mental disease or defect includes any abnormal condition of the mind which substantially affects mental or emotional processes and substantially impairs behavior controls. Thus the jury would consider testimony concerning the development, adaptation, and functioning of these processes and controls.

We emphasize that, since the question of whether the defendant has a disease or defect is ultimately for the triers of fact, obviously its resolution cannot be controlled by expert opinion. The jury must determine for itself, from all the testimony, lay and expert, whether the nature and degree of the disability are sufficient to es-

> *We emphasize that, since the question of whether the defendant has a disease or defect is ultimately for the triers of fact, obviously its resolution cannot be controlled by expert opinion.*

tablish a mental disease or defect as we have now defined those terms. What we have said, however, should in no way be construed to limit the latitude of expert testimony.

Medina v. California

505 U.S. 437 (1992)

Facts

In 1984, Teofilo Medina, Jr., held up two gas stations, a drive-in dairy, and a market; murdered three employees of those establishments; attempted to rob a fourth employee; and shot at two passers-by who attempted to follow his getaway car. He was apprehended less than one month after his crime spree began and was charged with a number of criminal offenses, including three counts of first-degree murder. Before trial, his counsel moved for a competency hearing on the grounds that he was unsure whether petitioner had the ability to participate in the criminal proceedings against him.

The court granted the motion pursuant to a state law forbidding a mentally incompetent defendant from being tried or punished. The statute established a presumption that the defendant is competent, and the party claiming incompetence bears the burden of proving by a preponderance of the evidence that the defendant is incompetent. The jury impaneled for the competency hearing found Medina competent to stand trial. A new jury was impaneled for the criminal trial, and Medina was subsequently convicted and sentenced to death.

Procedural History

The California Supreme Court affirmed, rejecting Medina's claim that the competency statute violated his right to due process by recognizing a presumption of competency and by placing the burden of proof on the defendant to refute that presumption. The U.S. Supreme Court granted *certiorari*.[1]

Issue

Does the Due Process Clause of the Fourteenth Amendment[2] permit a state to require a defendant who alleges incompetence to

---

[1] *certiorari*. A means of gaining appellate review.
[2] Due Process Clause; Fourteenth Amendment (Section 1). See Appendix B (p. 262).

stand trial to bear the burden of proving so by a preponderance of the evidence?

Holding

Yes. The Due Process Clause permits a state to require that a defendant claiming incompetence bear the burden of proving so by a preponderance of the evidence. The presumption of competence does not violate due process.

Analysis

The Supreme Court noted it had previously recognized that the power of a state to regulate procedures for carrying out its criminal laws - including the burdens of producing evidence and persuasion - is not subject to proscription under the Due Process Clause unless it "offends some principle of justice so rooted in the traditions and conscience of our people as to be ranked as fundamental." No settled tradition exists with regard to the proper allocation of the burden of proof in a competency proceeding. Further, contemporary practice demonstrates that there remains no settled view on where the burden should lie.

It has long been recognized that a defendant has a constitutional right not to be tried while legally incompetent. A state's failure to observe procedures adequate to protect a defendant's right not to be tried or convicted while incompetent deprives the defendant of due process rights to a fair trial. Once a state provides a defendant access to procedures for receiving a competency evaluation, however, there is no basis for holding that due process requires the state to assume the burden of protecting the defendant's constitutional right by persuading the trier of fact that the defendant is competent to stand trial. Traditionally, due process has required that only the most fundamental procedural safeguards be observed; more subtle balancing of society's interests against those of the accused has been left to legislatures. In practice, the state's allocation of the burden of proof to a defendant transgresses no recognized principle of "fundamental fairness."

Edited Excerpts[3]

Medina v. California

Supreme Court of the United States

---

[3] Readers are advised to quote only from the original published cases. See pages vii-viii.

Certiorari to the Supreme Court of California

505 U.S. 437

June 22, 1992

Kennedy, J., delivered the opinion of the Court, in which Rehnquist, C. J., and White, Scalia, and Thomas, JJ., joined. O'Connor, J., filed an opinion concurring in the judgment, in which Souter, J., joined. Blackmun, J., filed a dissenting opinion, in which Stevens, J., joined.

It is well established that the Due Process Clause of the Fourteenth Amendment prohibits the criminal prosecution of a defendant who is not competent to stand trial. The issue in this case is whether the Due Process Clause permits a State to require a defendant who alleges incompetence to stand trial to bear the burden of proving so by a preponderance of the evidence.

Under California law, "a person cannot be tried or adjudged to punishment while such person is mentally incompetent." A defendant is mentally incompetent "if, as a result of mental disorder or developmental disability, the defendant is unable to understand the nature of the criminal proceedings or to assist counsel in the conduct of a defense in a rational manner." The statute establishes a presumption that the defendant is competent, and the party claiming incompetence bears the burden of proving that the defendant is incompetent by a preponderance of the evidence. ("It shall be presumed that the defendant is mentally competent unless it is proved by a preponderance of the evidence that the defendant is mentally incompetent.")

The trial court granted the motion for a hearing and the preliminary issue of petitioner's competence to stand trial was tried to a jury. Over the course of the 6-day hearing, in addition to lay testimony, the jury heard conflicting expert testimony about petitioner's mental condition. The Supreme Court of California gives this summary: "Dr. Gold, a psychiatrist who knew defendant while he was in the Arizona prison system, testified that defendant was a paranoid schizophrenic and was incompetent to assist his attorney at trial. Dr. Echeandia, a clinical psychologist at the Orange County jail, doubted the accuracy of the schizo-

> **Reasonable minds may differ as to the wisdom of placing the burden of proof on the defendant.**

phrenia diagnosis, and could not express an opinion on defendant's competence to stand trial. Dr. Sharma, a psychiatrist, likewise expressed doubts regarding the schizophrenia diagnosis and leaned toward a finding of competence. Dr. Pierce, a psychologist, believed defendant was schizophrenic, with impaired memory and hallucinations, but nevertheless was competent to stand trial. Dr. Sakurai, a jail psychiatrist, opined that although defendant suffered from depression, he was competent, and that he may have been malingering. Dr. Sheffield, who treated defendant for knife wounds he incurred in jail, could give no opinion on the competency issue."

During the competency hearing, petitioner engaged in several verbal and physical outbursts. On one of these occasions, he overturned the counsel table. The trial court instructed the jury that "the defendant is presumed to be mentally competent and he has the burden of proving by a preponderance of the evidence that he is mentally incompetent as a result of mental disorder or developmental disability." The jury found petitioner com-

> **We cannot say that the allocation of the burden of proof to a criminal defendant to prove incompetence offends some fundamental principle of justice.**

petent to stand trial. A new jury was impaneled for the criminal trial, and petitioner entered pleas of not guilty and not guilty by reason of insanity. At the conclusion of the guilt phase, petitioner was found guilty of all three counts of first-degree murder and a number of lesser offenses. He moved to withdraw his insanity plea, and the trial court granted the motion. Two days later, however, petitioner moved to reinstate his insanity plea. Although his counsel expressed the view that reinstatement of the insanity plea was "tactically unsound," the trial court granted petitioner's motion. A sanity hearing was held, and the jury found that petitioner was sane at the time of the offenses. At the penalty phase, the jury found that the murders were premeditated and deliberate and returned a verdict of death. The trial court imposed the death penalty for the murder convictions and sentenced petitioner to a prison term for the remaining offenses.

On direct appeal to the California Supreme Court, petitioner did not challenge the standard of proof, but argued that the statute violated his right to due process by placing the burden of proof on him to establish that he was not competent to stand trial. In addition, he argued that that violates due process by establishing a presumption that a defendant is competent to stand trial unless proven otherwise. The court rejected both of these contentions.

Relying upon our decision in *Leland v. Oregon*, which rejected a due process challenge to an Oregon statute that required a criminal defendant to prove the defense of insanity beyond a reasonable doubt, the court observed that "the states ordinarily have great latitude to decide the proper placement of proof burdens." In its view, [the statute] "does not subject the defendant to hardship or oppression," because "one might reasonably expect that the defendant and his counsel would have better access than the People to the facts relevant to the court's competency inquiry." The court also rejected petitioner's argument that it is "irrational" to retain a presumption of competence after sufficient doubt has arisen as to a defendant's competence to warrant a hearing and "declined to hold as a matter of due process that such a presumption must be treated as a mere presumption affecting the burden of production, which disappears merely because a preliminary, often undefined and indefinite, 'doubt' has arisen that justifies further inquiry into the matter." We granted *certiorari* and now affirm.

Based on our review of the historical treatment of the burden of proof in competency proceedings, the operation of the challenged rule, and our precedents, we cannot say that the allocation of the burden of proof to a criminal defendant to prove incompetence "offends some principle of justice so rooted in the traditions and conscience of our people as to be ranked as fundamental." The rule that a criminal defendant who is incompetent should not be required to stand trial has deep roots in our common-law heritage. Blackstone[4] acknowledged that a defendant who became "mad" after the commission of an offense should not be arraigned for it "because he is not able to plead to it with that advice and caution that he ought," and "if he became 'mad' after pleading, he should not be tried, 'for how can he make his defense?' "

> *There are significant differences between a claim of incompetence and a plea of not guilty by reason of insanity.*

By contrast, there is no settled tradition on the proper allocation of the burden of proof in a proceeding to determine competence. Petitioner concedes that "the common law rule on this issue at the time the Constitution was adopted is not entirely clear." Early English authorities either express no view on the subject, for example, *King v. Steel,* stating that, once a jury had determined that the defendant was "mute by the visitation of God"

---

[4] Blackstone. Famous legal scholar.

(i.e., deaf and dumb) and not "mute of malice," there arose a "pre-sumption of ideotism" that the prosecution could rebut by demon-strating that the defendant had the capacity "to understand by signs and tokens."

Nineteenth century English decisions do not take a consistent position on the allocation of the burden of proof. American deci-sions dating from the turn of the century also express divergent views on the subject (e.g., *United States v. Chisolm*, defendant bears burden of raising a reasonable doubt as to competence; *State v. Helm*, burden on defendant to prove incompetence).

Contemporary practice, while of limited relevance to the due process inquiry, demonstrates that there remains no settled view of where the burden of proof should lie. The Federal Government and all 50 States have adopted procedures that address the issue of a defendant's competence to stand trial. Some States have en-acted statutes that, like [California's statute] place the burden of proof on the party raising the issue. A number of state courts have said that the burden of proof may be placed on the defen-dant to prove incompetence. Still other state courts have said that the burden rests with the prosecution.

Discerning no historical basis for concluding that the alloca-tion of the burden of proving incompetence to the defendant vio-lates due process, we turn to consider whether the rule trans-gresses any recognized principle of "fundamental fairness" in op-eration. Respondent argues that our decision in *Leland*, which upheld the right of the State to place on a defendant the burden of proving the defense of insanity beyond a reasonable doubt, compels the conclusion that [California's statute] is constitutional because, like a finding of insanity, a finding of incompetence has no necessary relationship to the elements of a crime, on which the State bears the burden of proof. This analogy is not convincing, because there are significant differences between a claim of in-competence and a plea of not guilty by reason of insanity.

In a competency hearing, the "emphasis is on the defendant's capacity to consult with counsel and to comprehend the proceed-ings, and this is by no means the same test as those which determine criminal responsibility at the time of the crime" (*Pate v. Robinson*). If a de-fendant is incompetent, due process considerations require suspension of the criminal trial until such time, if any, that the defendant regains the capac-

> *Due process does not require that every conceivable step be taken, at whatever cost, to eliminate the possibility of convicting an inno-cent person.*

ity to participate in his defense and understand the proceedings against him. See *Dusky v. United States.* The entry of a plea of not guilty by reason of insanity, by contrast, presupposes that the defendant is competent to stand trial and to enter a plea. Moreover, while the Due Process Clause affords an incompetent defendant the right not to be tried, we have not said that the Constitution requires the States to recognize the insanity defense.

Under California law, the allocation of the burden of proof to the defendant will affect competency determinations only in a narrow class of cases where the evidence is in equipoise; that is, where the evidence that a defendant is competent is just as strong as the evidence that he is incompetent. [We] recognize that a defendant has a constitutional right "not to be tried while legally incompetent," and that a State's "failure to observe procedures adequate to protect a defendant's right not to be tried or convicted while incompetent to stand trial deprives him of his due process right to a fair trial." Once a State provides a defendant access to procedures for making a competency evaluation, however, we perceive no basis for holding that due process further requires the State to assume the burden of vindicating the defendant's constitutional right by persuading the trier of fact that the defendant is competent to stand trial.

Petitioner relies upon federal- and state-court decisions which have said that the allocation of the burden of proof to the defendant in these circumstances is inconsistent with the rule of *Pate,* where we held that a defendant whose competence is in doubt cannot be deemed to have waived his right to a competency hearing. Because "it is contradictory to argue that a defendant may be incompetent, and yet knowingly or intelligently 'waive' his right to have the court determine his capacity to stand trial," it has been said that it is also "contradictory to argue that a defendant who may be incompetent should be presumed to possess sufficient intelligence that he will be able to adduce evidence of his incompetency which might otherwise be within his grasp."

In our view, the question whether a defendant whose competence is in doubt may waive his right to a competency hearing is quite different from the question whether the burden of proof may be placed on the defendant once a hearing is held. The rule announced in *Pate* was driven by our concern that it is impossible to say whether a defendant whose competence is in doubt has made a knowing and intelligent waiver of his right to a competency hearing. Once a competency hearing is held, however, the defendant is entitled to the assistance of counsel, for example, *Estelle v. Smith,* and psychiatric evidence is brought to bear on the question of the defendant's mental condition. Although an impaired defendant might be limited in his ability to assist counsel in demonstrating incompetence, the defendant's inability to assist counsel can, in and of itself, constitute probative evidence of incompetence, and defense counsel will often have the best-informed view of the defender's ability to participate in his defense. While reasonable minds may differ as to the wisdom of placing the burden of proof on the defendant in these circumstances, we believe that a State may take such factors into account in making judgments as to the allocation of the burden of proof, and we see no basis for concluding that placing the burden on the defendant violates the principle approved in *Pate*.

Petitioner argues that psychiatry is an inexact science, and that placing the burden of proof on the defendant violates due process because it requires the defendant to "bear the risk of being forced to stand trial as a result of an erroneous finding of competency." Our cases recognize that "the subtleties and nuances of psychiatric diagnosis render certainties virtually beyond reach in most situations," because "psychiatric diagnosis is to a large extent based on medical 'impressions' drawn from subjective analysis and filtered through the experience of the diagnostician" (*Addington v. Texas*). The Due Process Clause does not, however, require a State to adopt one procedure over another on the basis that it may produce results more favorable to the accused. ("Due process does not require that every conceivable step be taken, at whatever cost, to eliminate the possibility of convicting an innocent person," *Patterson v. New York*). Consistent with our precedents, it is enough that the State affords the criminal defendant on whose behalf a plea of incompetence is asserted a reasonable opportunity to demonstrate that he is not competent to stand trial.

Petitioner further contends that the burden of proof should be placed on the State because we have allocated the burden to the State on a variety of other issues that implicate a criminal defendant's constitutional rights. The decisions upon which petitioner relies, however, do not control the result here, because they involved situations where the government sought to introduce inculpatory evidence obtained by virtue of a waiver of, or in violation of, a defendant's constitutional rights. In such circumstances, allocating the burden of proof to the government furthers the objective of "deterring

> *Defense counsel will often have the best-informed view of the defendant's ability to participate in his defense.*

lawless conduct by police and prosecution." No such purpose is served by allocating the burden of proof to the government in a competency hearing.

In light of our determination that the allocation of the burden of proof to the defendant does not offend due process, it is not difficult to dispose of petitioner's challenge to the presumption of competence imposed by [California's statute]. Under California law, a defendant is required to make a threshold showing of incompetence before a hearing is required and, at the hearing, the defendant may be prevented from making decisions that are normally left to the discretion of a competent defendant. Petitioner argues that, once the trial court has expressed a doubt as to the defendant's competence, a hearing is held, and the defendant is deprived of his right to make determinations reserved to competent persons, it is irrational to retain the presumption that the defendant is competent.

In rejecting this contention below, the California Supreme Court observed that "the primary significance of the presumption of competence is to place on defendant (or the People, if they contest his competence) the burden of rebutting it" and that, "by its terms, the presumption of competence is one which affects the burden of proof." We see no reason to disturb the California Supreme Court's conclusion that, in essence, the challenged presumption is a restatement of the burden of proof, and it follows from what we have said that the presumption does not violate the Due Process Clause.

Nothing in today's decision is inconsistent with our longstanding recognition that the criminal trial of an incompetent defendant violates due process. Rather, our rejection of petitioner's challenge to [California's statute] is based on a determination that the California procedure is "constitutionally adequate" to guard against such results, and reflects our considered view that "traditionally, due process has required that only the most basic procedural safeguards be observed; more subtle balancing of society's interests against those of the accused has been left to the legislative branch."

The judgment of the Supreme Court of California is Affirmed.

Justice O'Connor, With Whom Justice Souter Joins, Concurring in the Judgment

After balancing the equities in this case, I agree with the Court that the burden of proof may constitutionally rest on the defendant. As the dissent points out, the competency determination is based largely on the testimony of psychiatrists. The main concern of the prosecution, of course, is that a defendant will feign incompetence in order to avoid trial. If the burden of proving competence rests on the government, a defendant will have less incentive to cooper-

> **The main concern of the prosecution, of course, is that a defendant will feign incompetence in order to avoid trial. (O'Connor, Concurring)**

ate in psychiatric investigations, because an inconclusive examination will benefit the defense, not the prosecution. A defendant may also be less cooperative in making available friends or family who might have information about the defendant's mental state. States may therefore decide that a more complete picture of a defendant's competence will be obtained if the defense has the incentive to produce all the evidence in its possession. The potentially greater overall access to information provided by placing the burden of proof on the defense may outweigh the danger that, in close cases, a marginally incompetent defendant is brought to trial. Unlike the requirement of a hearing or a psychiatric examination, placing the burden of proof on the government will not necessarily increase the reliability of the proceedings. The equities here, then, do not weigh so much in petitioner's favor as to rebut the presumption of constitutionality that the historical toleration of procedural variation creates.

Justice Blackmun, With Whom Justice Stevens Joins, Dissenting

Teofilo Medina, Jr., may have been mentally incompetent when the State of California convicted him and sentenced him to death. One psychiatrist testified he was incompetent. Another psychiatrist and a psychologist testified he was not. Several other experts testified but did not express an opinion on competence. Instructed to presume that petitioner Medina was competent, the jury returned a finding of competence. For all we know, the jury was entirely undecided. I do not believe a Constitution that forbids the trial and conviction of an incompetent person tolerates the trial and conviction of a person about whom the evidence of competency is so equivocal and unclear. I dissent.

The right of a criminal defendant to be tried only if competent is "fundamental to an adversary system of justice." The Due Process Clause forbids the trial and conviction of persons incapable of defending themselves - persons lacking the capacity to understand the nature and object of the proceedings against them, to consult with counsel, and to assist in preparing their defense.

The right to be tried while competent is the foundational right for the effective exercise of a defendant's other rights in a criminal trial. "Competence to stand trial is rudimentary, for upon it depends the main part of those rights deemed essential to a fair trial, including the right to effective assistance of counsel, the rights to summon, to confront, and to cross-examine witnesses, and the right to testify on one's own behalf or to remain silent without penalty for doing so" (*Riggins v. Nevada*). In the words of Professor Morris, one of the world's leading criminologists, incompetent persons "are not really present at trial; they may not be able properly to play the role of an accused person, to recall relevant events, to produce evidence and witnesses, to testify effectively on their own behalf, to help confront hostile witnesses, and to project to the trier of facts a sense of their innocence."

This Court's cases are clear that the right to be tried while competent is so critical a prerequisite to the criminal process that "state procedures must be adequate to protect this right." In other words, the Due Process Clause does not simply forbid the State to try to convict a person who is incompetent. It also demands adequate anticipatory, protective proce-

> **Because the Due Process Clause is not the Some Process Clause, I remain convinced that it requires careful balancing of the individual and governmental interests at stake to determine what process is due. (Blackmun, dissenting)**

dures to minimize the risk that an incompetent person will be convicted.

This Court expressly has recognized that one of the required procedural protections is "further inquiry" or a hearing when there is a sufficient doubt raised about a defendant's competency. In my view, then, the only question before the Court in this case is whether - as with the right to a hearing - placing the burden of proving competence on the State is necessary to protect adequately the underlying due process right. I part company with the Court today, because I believe the answer to that question is in the affirmative.

As an initial matter, I believe the Court's approach to this case effectively asks and answers the wrong doctrinal question. Under *Drope* and *Pate*, it need decide only whether a procedure imposing the burden of proof upon the defendant is "adequate" to protect the constitutional prohibition against trial of incompetent persons.

The Court, however, chooses the *Patterson* path, announcing that there is no violation of due process unless placing the burden of proof of incompetency upon the defendant "offends some principle of justice so rooted in the traditions and conscience of our people as to be ranked as fundamental." Separating the primary right (the right not to be tried while incompetent) from the subsidiary right (the right not to bear the burden of proof of incompetency), the Court acknowledges the primary right to be fundamental in "our common-law heritage," but determines the subsidiary right to be without a "settled tradition" deserving of constitutional protection. This approach is mistaken, because it severs two integrally related procedural rights that cannot be examined meaningfully in isolation. The protections of the Due Process Clause, to borrow the second Justice Harlan's words, are simply not "a series of isolated points pricked" out in terms of their most specific level of historic generality. Had the Court taken the same historical-categorical approach in *Pate* and *Drope*, it would not have recognized that a defendant has a right to a competency hearing, for in neither of those cases was there any showing that the mere denial of a hearing where there is doubt about competency offended any deeply rooted traditions of the American people.

The Court points out that the defendant is already entitled to the assistance of counsel and to a psychiatric evaluation. It suggests as well that defense counsel will have "the best-informed view" of the defendant's ability to assist in his defense. Accordingly, the Court concludes: "It is enough that the State affords the criminal defendant on whose behalf a plea of incompetence is asserted a reasonable opportunity to demonstrate that he is not competent to stand trial."

I am perplexed that the Court, while recognizing "the careful balance that the Constitution strikes between liberty and order," intimates that the apparent "expertise" of the States in criminal procedure and the "centuries of common-law tradition" of the "criminal process" warrant less than careful balancing in favor of "substantial deference to legislative judgments." Because the Due Process Clause is not the Some Process Clause, I remain convinced that it requires careful balancing of the individual and governmental interests at stake to determine what process is due.

> *Yet in cases where the evidence is inconclusive, a defendant bearing the burden of proof of his own incompetency now will still be subjected to trial. (Blackmun, dissenting)*

I believe that requiring a possibly incompetent person to carry the burden of proving that he is incompetent cannot be called "adequate," within the meaning of the decisions in *Pate* and *Drope*, to protect a defendant's right to be tried only while competent. Equally weighty concerns warrant imposing the burden of proof upon the State here.

"In all kinds of litigation it is plain that where the burden of proof lies may be decisive of the outcome" (*Speiser v. Randall*). To be sure, the requirement of a hearing (once there is a threshold doubt as to competency) and the provision for a psychiatric evaluation do ensure at least some protection against the trial of incompetent persons. Yet in cases where the evidence is inconclusive, a defendant bearing the burden of proof of his own incompetency now will still be subjected to trial. In my view, this introduces a systematic and unacceptably high risk that persons will be tried and convicted who are unable to follow or participate in the proceedings determining their fate. I, therefore, cannot agree with the Court that "reasonable minds may differ as to the wisdom of placing the burden of proof" on likely incompetent defendants.

The Court suggests that "defense counsel will often have the best-informed view of the defendant's ability to participate in his defense." There are at least three good reasons, however, to doubt the Court's confidence. First, while the defendant is in custody, the State itself obviously has the most direct, unfettered access to him and is in the best position to observe his behavior. In the present case, Medina was held before trial in the Orange County jail system for more than a year and a half prior to his competency hearing. During the months immediately preceding the competency hearing, he was placed several times for extended periods in a padded cell for treatment and observation by prison psychiatric personnel. While Medina was in the padded cell, prison personnel observed his behavior every 15 minutes.

Second, a competency determination is primarily a medical and psychiatric determination. Competency determinations by and large turn on the testimony of psychiatric experts, not lawyers. While the testimony of psychiatric experts may be far from infallible, it is the experts and not the lawyers who are credited as the "best informed," and most able to gauge a defendant's ability to understand and participate in the legal proceedings affecting him.

Third, even assuming that defense counsel has the "best-informed view" of the defendant's competency, the lawyer's view will likely have no outlet in, or effect on, the competency determination. Unlike the testimony of medical specialists or lay wit-witnesses, the testimony of defense counsel is far more likely to be discounted by the factfinder as self-interested and biased. Defense counsel

> *Competency determinations by and large turn on the testimony of psychiatric experts, not lawyers. (Blackmun, dissenting)*

may also be discouraged in the first place from testifying for fear of abrogating an ethical responsibility or the attorney-client privilege. By way of example from the case at hand, it should come as little surprise that neither of Medina's two attorneys was among the dozens of persons testifying during the six days of competency proceedings in this case.

Like many psychological inquiries, competency evaluations are "in the present state of the mental sciences at best a hazardous guess however conscientious." This unavoidable uncertainty expands the range of cases where the factfinder will conclude the evidence is in equipoise. The Court, however, dismisses this concern on grounds that "due process does not require that every conceivable step be taken, at whatever cost, to eliminate the possibility of convicting an innocent person." Yet surely the Due Process Clause requires some conceivable steps be taken to eliminate the risk of erroneous convictions. I search in vain for any guiding principle in the Court's analysis that determines when the risk of a wrongful conviction happens to be acceptable and when it does not.

The allocation of the burden of proof reflects a societal judgment about how the risk of error should be distributed between litigants. This Court has said it well before: "The individual should not be asked to share equally with society the risk of error when the possible injury to the individual is significantly greater than any possible harm to the state" (*Addington*). The costs to the State of bearing the burden of proof of competency are not at all prohibitive. The Court ac-knowledges that several States already bear the burden, and that the allocation of the burden of proof will make a difference "only in a narrow class of cases where the

> *Like many psychological inquiries, competency evaluations are "in the present state of the mental sciences at best a hazardous guess however conscientious." (Blackmun, dissenting)*

evidence is in equipoise." In those few difficult cases, the State should bear the burden of remitting the defendant for further psychological observation to ensure that he is competent to defend himself. In the narrow class of cases where the evidence is in equipoise, the State can reasonably expect that it will speedily be able to return the defendant for trial.

Just this Term the Court reaffirmed that the Due Process Clause prevents the States from taking measures that undermine the defendant's right to be tried while fully aware and able to defend himself. In *Riggins*, the Court reversed on due process grounds the conviction of a defendant subjected to the forcible administration of antipsychotic drugs during his trial. Rejecting the dissent's insistence that actual prejudice be shown, the Court found it to be "clearly possible" that the medications affected the defendant's "ability to follow the proceedings, or the substance of his communication with counsel." I consider it no less likely that petitioner Medina was tried and sentenced to death while effectively unable to defend himself. That is why I do not share the Court's remarkable confidence that "nothing in today's decision is inconsistent with our longstanding recognition that the criminal trial of an incompetent defendant violates due process." I do not believe the constitutional prohibition against convicting incompetent persons remains "fundamental" if the State is at liberty to go forward with a trial when the evidence of competency is inconclusive.

Accordingly, I dissent.

Cooper v. Oklahoma

517 U.S. 348 (1996)

Facts

In 1989, Byron Keith Cooper was charged with killing an 86-year-old man during the course of a burglary. The issue of Cooper's competence was raised before and during his trial. On five separate occasions, a judge considered whether Cooper had the ability to understand the charges against him and to assist defense counsel. On each occasion the judge concluded the defendant was competent based on the standard of proof to demonstrate competency in the state of Oklahoma. Under Oklahoma law at that time, the defendant in a criminal prosecution was presumed to be competent to stand trial unless able to prove incompetence by clear and convincing evidence. Under that standard, a defendant could have been put to trial even though he or she is more likely than not incompetent.

An Oklahoma jury found Cooper guilty of first-degree murder and recommended punishment by death. The trial court imposed the death penalty. The Oklahoma Court of Criminal Appeals affirmed the conviction and sentence.

Issue

Does Oklahoma's procedural rule allowing the state to try a defendant who is more likely than not incompetent violate due process under the Fourteenth Amendment?[1]

Holding

Oklahoma's procedural rule allowing the state to try a defendant who is more likely than not incompetent violates due process. The clear and convincing standard of proof to determine competency to proceed is unconstitutional.

---

[1] Due Process Clause of the Fourteenth Amendment (Section 1). See Appendix B (p. 262).

Analysis

Oklahoma's heightened standard is not necessary to protect the state's interest in prompt and orderly disposition of criminal cases. An erroneous determination of competence has dire consequences for a defendant who has already demonstrated that he is more likely than not incompetent, threatening the basic fairness of the trial itself. Difficulty in ascertaining whether a defendant is incompetent or malingering may make it appropriate to place the burden of proof on a defendant, but it does not justify the additional onus of an especially high standard of proof.

Although it is normally within a state's power to establish the procedures through which its laws are given effect, the power to regulate procedural burdens is subject to proscription under the Due Process Clause when the procedures do not sufficiently protect a fundamental constitutional right. Here, the fundamental right not to stand trial while incompetent was not sufficiently protected.

Edited Excerpts[2]

Cooper v. Oklahoma

United States Supreme Court

Certiorari to the Court of Criminal Appeals of Oklahoma

517 U.S. 348

April 16, 1996

Stevens, J., Delivered the Opinion for a Unanimous Court

In 1989 petitioner was charged with the brutal killing of an 86-year-old man in the course of a burglary. After an Oklahoma jury found him guilty of first-degree murder and recommended punishment by death, the trial court imposed the death penalty. The Oklahoma Court of Criminal Appeals affirmed the conviction and sentence.

---

[2] Readers are advised to quote only from the original published cases. See pages vii-viii.

Petitioner's competence was the focus of significant attention both before and during his trial. On five separate occasions a judge considered whether petitioner had the ability to understand the charges against him and to assist defense counsel. On the first occasion, a pretrial judge relied on the opinion of a clinical psychologist employed by the State to find petitioner incompetent. Based on that determination, he committed petitioner to a state mental health facility for treatment.

Upon petitioner's release from the hospital some three months later, the trial judge heard testimony concerning petitioner's competence from two state-employed psychologists. These experts expressed conflicting opinions regarding petitioner's ability to participate in his defense. The judge resolved the dispute against petitioner, ordering him to proceed to trial.

At the close of the pretrial hearing held one week before the trial was scheduled to begin, the lead defense attorney raised the issue of petitioner's competence for a third time. Counsel advised the court that petitioner was behaving oddly and refusing to communicate with him. Defense counsel opined that it would be a serious matter "if he's not faking." After listening to

> *Normal is like us. Anybody that's not like us is not normal, so I don't think normal is a proper definition that we are to use with incompetence. (Trial judge)*

counsel's concerns, however, the judge declined to revisit his earlier determination that petitioner was competent to stand trial.

Petitioner's competence was addressed a fourth time on the first day of trial, when petitioner's bizarre behavior prompted the court to conduct a further competency hearing at which the judge observed petitioner and heard testimony from several lay witnesses, a third psychologist, and petitioner himself.[3] The expert concluded that petitioner was presently incompetent and unable to communicate effectively with counsel, but that he could probably achieve competence within six weeks if treated aggressively. While stating that he did not dispute the psychologist's diagnosis, the trial judge ruled against petitioner. In so holding, however, the court voiced uncertainty: "Well, I think I've used the expression in the past that normal is like us. Anybody that's not like us is not normal, so I don't think normal is a proper definition that

---

[3] During the hearing petitioner, who had refused to change out of prison overalls for the trial because the proffered clothes were "burning" him, talked to himself and to an imaginary "spirit" who petitioner claimed gave him counsel. On the witness stand petitioner expressed fear that the lead defense attorney wanted to kill him.

we are to use with incompetence. My shirtsleeve opinion of Mr. Cooper is that he's not normal. Now, to say he's not competent is something else. I think it's going to take smarter people than me to make a decision here. I'm going to say that I don't believe he has carried the burden by clear and convincing evidence of his incompetency and I'm going to say we're going to trial."

Incidents that occurred during the trial,[4] as well as the sordid history of petitioner's childhood that was recounted during the sentencing phase of the proceedings, were consistent with the conclusions expressed by the expert. In a final effort to protect his client's interests, defense counsel moved for a mistrial or a renewed investigation into petitioner's competence. After the court summarily denied these motions, petitioner was convicted and sentenced to death.

In the Court of Criminal Appeals, petitioner contended that Oklahoma's presumption of competence, combined with its statutory requirement that a criminal defendant establish incompetence by clear and convincing evidence placed such an onerous burden on him as to violate his right to due process of law. The appellate court rejected this argument. After noting that it can be difficult to determine whether a defendant

> **The Court held that the truly incompetent criminal defendant, through his attorneys and experts, can prove incompetency with relative ease.**

is malingering, given "the inexactness and uncertainty attached to competency proceedings," the court held that the standard was justified because the "State has great interest in assuring its citizens a thorough and speedy judicial process," and because a "truly incompetent criminal defendant, through his attorneys and experts, can prove incompetency with relative ease." We granted *certiorari* to review the Court of Criminal Appeals' conclusion that application of the clear and convincing evidence standard does not violate due process.

Our recent decision in *Medina v. California* establishes that a State may presume that the defendant is competent and require him to shoulder the burden of proving his incompetence by a preponderance of the evidence. [Early English cases] suggest that traditional practice required the jury to determine whether the defendant was "more likely than not" incompetent. Nothing in the jury instructions of these cases will bear the interpretation of a

---

[4] Petitioner did not communicate with or sit near defense counsel during the trial. Through much of the proceedings he remained in prison overalls, crouching in the fetal position and talking to himself.

clear and convincing standard. Modern English authority confirms our interpretations of these early cases as applying a preponderance standard.

Likewise, we are aware of no decisional law from this country suggesting that any State employed Oklahoma's standard until quite recently. The question we address today is quite different from the question posed in *Medina*. Petitioner's claim requires us to consider whether a State may proceed with a criminal trial after the defendant has demonstrated that he is more likely than not incompetent. Oklahoma does not contend that it may require the defendant to prove incompetence beyond a reasonable doubt. The State maintains, however, that the clear and convincing standard provides a reasonable accommodation of the opposing interests of the State and the defendant. We are persuaded, by both traditional and modern practice and the importance of the constitutional interest at stake, that the State's argument must be rejected.

Contemporary practice demonstrates that the vast majority of jurisdictions remain persuaded that the heightened standard of proof imposed on the accused in Oklahoma is not necessary to vindicate the State's interest in prompt and orderly disposition of criminal cases. Only 4 of the 50 States presently require the criminal defendant to prove his incompetence by clear and convincing evidence. None of the remaining 46 jurisdictions imposes such a heavy burden on the defendant. Indeed, a number of States place no burden on the defendant at all, but rather require the prosecutor to prove the defendant's competence to stand trial once a question about competency has been credibly raised. The situation is no different in federal court. Congress has directed that the accused in a federal prosecution must prove incompetence by a preponderance of the evidence.

The near-uniform application of a standard that is more protective of the defendant's rights than Oklahoma's clear and convincing evidence rule supports our conclusion that the heightened standard offends a principle of justice that is deeply "rooted in the traditions and conscience of our people." We turn next to a consideration of whether the rule exhibits "funda-

> *An erroneous determination of competence threatens a "fundamental component of our criminal justice system" - the basic fairness of the trial itself.*

mental fairness in operation." Contemporary and historical procedures are fully consistent with our evaluation of the risks inherent in Oklahoma's practice of requiring the defendant to prove incompetence by clear and convincing evidence. In *Addington v. Texas* we explained that: "The function of a standard of proof, as that concept is embodied in the Due Process Clause[5] and in the realm of fact finding, is to 'instruct the factfinder concerning the degree of confidence our society thinks he should have in the correctness of factual conclusions for a particular type of adjudication.' "

Far from "jealously guarding" an incompetent criminal defendant's fundamental right not to stand trial, Oklahoma's practice of requiring the defendant to prove incompetence by clear and convincing evidence imposes a significant risk of an erroneous determination that the defendant is competent. For the defendant, the consequences of an erroneous determination of competence are dire. Because he lacks the ability to communicate effectively with counsel, he may be unable to exercise other "rights deemed essential to a fair trial" (*Riggins v. Nevada*). After making the "profound" choice whether to plead guilty, the defendant who proceeds to trial "will ordinarily have to decide whether to waive his 'privilege against compulsory self-incrimination' by taking the witness stand; if the option is available, he may have to decide whether to waive his 'right to trial by jury,' and, in consultation with counsel, he may have to decide whether to waive his 'right to confront his accusers,' by declining to cross-examine witnesses for the prosecution" (*Boykin v. Alabama*). With the assistance of counsel, the defendant also is called upon to make myriad smaller decisions concerning the course of his defense. The importance of these rights and decisions demonstrates that an erroneous determination of competence threatens a "fundamental component of our criminal justice system" - the basic fairness of the trial itself.

The Oklahoma Court of Criminal Appeals correctly observed that the "inexactness and uncertainty" that characterize competency proceedings may make it difficult to determine whether a defendant is incompetent or malingering. We presume, however, that it is unusual for even the most artful malingerer to feign incompetence successfully for a period of time while under professional care. In this regard it is worth reiterating that only four jurisdictions currently consider it necessary to impose on the criminal defendant the burden of proving incompetence by clear and convincing evidence. Moreover, there is no reason to believe that the art of dissimulation is new. Eighteenth and nineteenth century courts, for example, warned jurors charged with making

---

[5] Due Process Clause of the Fourteenth Amendment. See Appendix B (p. 262).

competency determinations that "there may be great fraud in this matter" and that "it would be a reproach to justice if a guilty man postponed his trial upon a feigned condition of mind, as to his inability to aid in his defense." Although they recognized this risk, the early authorities did not resort to a heightened burden of proof in competency proceedings.

A heightened standard does not decrease the risk of error, but simply reallocates that risk between the parties. In cases in which competence is at issue, we perceive no sound basis for allocating to the criminal defendant the large share of the risk which accompanies a clear and convincing evidence standard. We assume that questions of competence will arise in a range of cases including not only those in which one side will prevail with relative ease, but also those in which it is more likely than not that the defendant is incompetent but the evidence is insufficiently strong to satisfy a clear and convincing standard. While important state interests are unquestionably at stake, in these latter cases the defendant's fundamental right to be tried only while competent outweighs the State's interest in the efficient operation of its criminal justice system.

Finally, Oklahoma suggests that our decision in *Addington*, in which we held that due process requires a clear and convincing standard of proof in an involuntary civil commitment proceeding, supports imposition of such a rule in competency proceedings. The argument is unpersuasive because commitment and competency proceedings address entirely different substantive issues. More importantly, our decision today is in complete accord with the

> *Because Oklahoma's procedural rule allows the State to put to trial a defendant who is more likely than not incompetent, the rule is incompatible with the dictates of due process.*

basis for our ruling in *Addington*. [Such] cases concern the proper protection of fundamental rights in circumstances in which the State proposes to take drastic action against an individual. The requirement that the grounds for civil commitment be shown by clear and convincing evidence protects the individual's fundamental interest in liberty. The *prohibition* against requiring the criminal defendant to demonstrate incompetence by clear and convincing evidence safeguards the fundamental right not to stand trial while incompetent. Because Oklahoma's procedural rule allows the State to put to trial a defendant who is more likely than not incompetent, the rule is incompatible with the dictates of due process.

Godinez v. Moran

509 U.S. 389 (1993)

Facts

After defendant Richard Allen Moran pled not guilty to three counts of murder, the trial court ordered examinations by two psychiatrists. Both concluded that Moran was competent to stand trial. The state thereafter announced its intention to seek the death penalty. Two and one-half months after the psychiatric evaluations, Moran informed the court he wished to discharge his attorneys and change his plea to guilty, reportedly to prevent the presentation of mitigating evidence at his sentencing. The trial court accepted the waiver of counsel and the guilty plea, having found that Moran understood the nature of the charges against him and was able to assist in his defense. The court also explicitly found that Moran had "knowingly and intelligently" waived his right to counsel and that his guilty plea was "freely and voluntarily" given. Moran was ultimately sentenced to death for two of the murders.

Procedural History

Moran sought post-conviction relief in state court, claiming he had been mentally incompetent to represent himself. Following an evidentiary hearing, the trial court rejected Moran's claim. The state supreme court dismissed Moran's appeal, and the U.S. Supreme Court denied *certiorari*.[1]

Moran then filed a *habeas petition*[2] in federal district court. The district court denied the petition. The Court of Appeals for the Ninth Circuit reversed, holding that due process required the trial court to hold a competency hearing before accepting Moran's decision to waive counsel and plead guilty, and that the trial court's post-conviction ruling was premised on the wrong legal standard of competency. The Court of Appeals held that competency to waive constitutional rights requires a higher level of mental functioning than that required to stand trial (i.e., that a defendant is competent to waive counsel or plead guilty only if

---

[1] *certiorari.* A means of gaining appellate review.
[2] *habeas petition.* Request to review the legality of an individual's custody.

possessing "the capacity for 'reasoned choice' among the alternatives available to him"). The U.S. Supreme Court then granted *certiorari*.

Issue

Is the competency standard for pleading guilty or waiving the right to counsel higher than the competency standard for standing trial?

Holding

A higher standard of competency is not required to plead guilty or to waive the right to counsel. The *Dusky* standard for competency to stand trial is the same competency standard required for a defendant to plead guilty or to waive the right to assistance of counsel.

Analysis

The Court reasoned that all criminal defendants may be required to make important decisions once criminal proceedings have been initiated. The decision to plead guilty is no more complicated than the sum total of decisions a defendant may be called upon to make during the course of a trial. Similarly, there is no reason to believe that the decision to waive counsel requires an appreciably higher level of mental functioning than the decision to waive other constitutional rights. In addition to a finding of competency, however, a trial court must determine that a defendant's waiver of constitutional rights is *knowing and voluntary*. The purpose of this "knowing and voluntary" inquiry is to determine (1) whether the defendant actually does understand the significance and consequences of the decision, and (2) whether the decision is uncoerced.

Edited Excerpts[3]

Salvador Godinez, Warden, Petitioner v. Richard Allen Moran

Supreme Court of the United States

---

[3] Readers are advised to quote only from the original published cases. See pages vii-viii.

Certiorari to the United States Court of
Appeals for the Ninth Circuit

509 U.S. 389

June 24, 1993

Thomas, J., delivered the opinion of the Court, in which
Rehnquist, C.J., and White, O'Connor, and Souter, JJ.,
joined, and in parts of which Scalia and Kennedy, JJ.,
joined. Kennedy, J., filed an opinion concurring in part
and concurring in the judgment, in which Scalia, J.,
joined. Blackmun, J., filed a dissenting opinion, in which
Stevens, J., joined.

On August 2, 1984, in the early hours of the morning, respondent entered the Red Pearl Saloon in Las Vegas, Nevada, and shot the bartender and a patron four times each with an automatic pistol. He then walked behind the bar and removed the cash register. Nine days later, respondent arrived at the apartment of his former wife and opened fire on her; five of his seven shots hit their target. Respondent then shot himself in the abdo-

> **While the decision to plead guilty is undeniably a profound one, it is no more complicated than the sum total of decisions that a defendant may be called upon to make during the course of a trial.**

men and attempted, without success, to slit his wrists. Of the four victims of respondent's gunshots, only respondent himself survived. On August 13, respondent summoned police to his hospital bed and confessed to the killings. After respondent pleaded not guilty to three counts of first-degree murder, the trial court ordered that he be examined by a pair of psychiatrists, both of whom concluded that he was competent to stand trial. The State thereafter announced its intention to seek the death penalty. On November 28, 1984, 2½ months after the psychiatric evaluations, respondent again appeared before the trial court. At this time, respondent informed the court that he wished to discharge his attorneys and change his pleas to guilty. The reason for the request, according to respondent, was to prevent the presentation of mitigating evidence at his sentencing. On the basis of the psychiatric reports, the trial court found that respondent "is competent in that he knew the nature and quality of his acts, had the capacity to determine right from wrong; that he understands the nature of the criminal charges against him and is able to assist in his defense of such charges, or against the pronouncement of the judgment thereafter; that he knows the consequences of entering a plea of guilty to the charges; and that he can intelligently and knowingly waive his constitutional right to assistance of an attorney."

The court advised respondent that he had a right both to the assistance of counsel and to self-representation, warned him of the "dangers and disadvantages" of self-representation, inquired into his understanding of the proceedings and his awareness of his rights, and asked why he had chosen to represent himself. It then accepted respondent's waiver of counsel. The court also accepted respondent's guilty pleas, but not before it had determined that respondent was not pleading guilty in response to threats or promises, that he understood the nature of the charges against him and the consequences of pleading guilty, that he was aware of the rights he was giving up, and that there was a factual basis for the pleas. The trial court explicitly found that respondent was "knowingly and intelligently" waiving his right to the assistance of counsel, and that his guilty pleas were "freely and voluntarily" given.

On January 21, 1985, a three-judge court sentenced respondent to death for each of the murders. The Supreme Court of Nevada affirmed respondent's sentences for the Red Pearl Saloon murders, but reversed his sentence for the murder of his ex-wife and remanded for imposition of a life sentence without the possibility of parole. On July 30, 1987, respondent filed a petition for post-conviction relief in state court. Following an evidentiary hearing, the

> **We reject the notion that competence to plead guilty or to waive the right to counsel must be measured by a standard that is higher than (or even different from) the Dusky standard.**

trial court rejected respondent's claim that he was "mentally incompetent to represent himself," concluding that "the record clearly shows that he was examined by two psychiatrists, both of whom declared him competent." The Supreme Court of Nevada dismissed respondent's appeal, and we denied *certiorari*. Respondent then filed a *habeas* petition in the United States District Court for the District of Nevada. The District Court denied the petition, but the Ninth Circuit reversed. The Court of Appeals concluded that the "record in this case" should have led the trial court to "entertain a good faith doubt about respondent's competency to make a voluntary, knowing, and intelligent waiver of constitutional rights," and that the Due Process Clause therefore "required the court to hold a hearing to evaluate and determine respondent's competency before it accepted his decision to discharge counsel and change his pleas." Rejecting petitioner's argument that the trial court's error was "cured by the post-conviction hearing," and that the competency determination that followed the hearing was entitled to deference under [federal statute], the Court of Appeals held that "the state court's post-conviction ruling was premised on the wrong legal standard of competency." "Competency to waive constitutional rights," according to the Court of Appeals, "requires a higher level of mental functioning than that required to stand trial"; while a defendant is competent to stand trial if he has "a rational and factual understanding of the proceedings and is capable of assisting his counsel," a defendant is competent to waive counsel or plead guilty only if he has "the capacity for 'reasoned choice' among the alternatives available to him." The Court of Appeals determined that the trial court had "erroneously applied the standard for evaluating competency to stand trial, instead of the correct 'reasoned choice' standard," and further concluded that, when examined "in light of the correct legal standard," the record did not support a finding that respondent was "mentally capable of the reasoned choice required for a valid waiver of constitutional rights." Whether the competency standard for pleading guilty or waiving the right to counsel is higher than the competency standard for standing trial is a question that has divided the Federal Courts of Appeals and state courts of last resort. We granted *certiorari* to resolve the conflict.

A criminal defendant may not be tried unless he is competent (*Pate v. Robinson*), and he may not waive his right to counsel or plead guilty unless he does so "competently and intelligently" (*Johnson v. Zerbst*). In *Dusky*, we held that the standard for competence to stand trial is whether the defendant has "sufficient present ability to consult with his lawyer with a reasonable degree of rational under-

> **If the Dusky standard is adequate for defendants who plead not guilty, it is necessarily adequate for those who plead guilty.**

standing" and has "a rational as well as factual understanding of the proceedings against him." While we have described the standard for competence to stand trial, however, we have never expressly articulated a standard for competence to plead guilty or to waive the right to the assistance of counsel.

Relying in large part upon our decision in *Westbrook v. Arizona*, the Ninth Circuit adheres to the view that the competency standard for pleading guilty or waiving the right to counsel is higher than the competency standard for standing trial. In *Westbrook*, a two-paragraph *per curiam*[4] opinion, we vacated the lower court's judgment affirming the petitioner's conviction, because there had been "a hearing on the issue of the petitioner's competence to stand trial," but "no hearing or inquiry into the issue of his competence to waive his constitutional right to the assistance of counsel." The Ninth Circuit has reasoned that the "clear implication" of *Westbrook* is that the *Dusky* formulation is not "a high enough standard" for determining whether a defendant is competent to waive a constitutional right.[5] We think the Ninth Circuit has read too much into *Westbrook*, and we think it errs in applying two different competency standards.

The standard adopted by the Ninth Circuit is whether a defendant who seeks to plead guilty or waive counsel has the capacity for "reasoned choice" among the alternatives available to him. How this standard is different from (much less higher than) the *Dusky* standard - whether the defendant has a "rational understanding" of the proceedings - is not readily apparent to us. But even assuming that there is some meaningful distinction between the capacity for "reasoned choice" and a "rational understanding" of the proceedings, we reject the notion that competence to plead guilty or to waive the right to counsel must be measured by a standard that is higher than (or even different from) the *Dusky* standard.

We begin with the guilty plea. A defendant who stands trial is likely to be presented with choices that entail relinquishment of the same rights that are relinquished by a defendant who pleads guilty: He will ordinarily have to decide whether to waive his "privilege against compulsory self-incrimination" (*Boykin v. Alabama*), by taking the witness stand; if the option is available, he may have to decide whether to waive his "right to trial by jury," and, in consultation with counsel, he may have to decide whether to waive his "right to confront his accusers," by declining to cross-examine witnesses for the prosecution. A defendant who pleads not guilty, moreover, faces still other

> **There is a heightened standard for pleading guilty and for waiving the right to counsel, but it is not a heightened standard of competence.**

---

[4] *per curiam.* By the court, no single opinion writer identified.

[5] A criminal defendant waives three constitutional rights when he pleads guilty: the privilege against self-incrimination, the right to a jury trial, and the right to confront one's accusers (*Boykin v. Alabama*).

strategic choices: In consultation with his attorney, he may be called upon to decide, among other things, whether (and how) to put on a defense and whether to raise one or more affirmative defenses. In sum, all criminal defendants - not merely those who plead guilty - may be required to make important decisions once criminal proceedings have been initiated. And while the decision to plead guilty is undeniably a profound one, it is no more complicated than the sum total of decisions that a defendant may be called upon to make during the course of a trial. (The decision to plead guilty is also made over a shorter period of time, without the distraction and burden of a trial.) This being so, we can conceive of no basis for demanding a higher level of competence for those defendants who choose to plead guilty. If the *Dusky* standard is adequate for defendants who plead not guilty, it is necessarily adequate for those who plead guilty.

Nor do we think that a defendant who waives his right to the assistance of counsel must be more competent than a defendant who does not, since there is no reason to believe that the decision to waive counsel requires an appreciably higher level of mental functioning than the decision to waive other constitutional rights. Respondent suggests that a higher competency standard is necessary because a defendant who represents himself "must have greater powers of comprehension, judgment, and reason than would be necessary to stand trial with the aid of an attorney." But this argument has a flawed premise; the competence that is required of a defendant seeking to waive his right to counsel is the competence to *waive the right*, not the competence to represent himself. In *Faretta v. California*, we held that a defendant choosing self-representation must do so "competently and intelligently," but we made it clear that the defendant's "technical legal knowledge" is "not relevant" to the determination whether he is competent to waive his right to counsel, and we emphasized that although the defendant "may conduct his own defense ultimately to his own detriment, his choice must be honored." Thus, while "it

> *While psychiatrists and scholars may find it useful to classify the various kinds and degrees of competence, the Due Process Clause does not impose these additional requirements.*

is undeniable that in most criminal prosecutions defendants could better defend with counsel's guidance than by their own unskilled efforts," a criminal defendant's ability to represent himself has no bearing upon his competence to choose self-representation.

A finding that a defendant is competent to stand trial, however, is not all that is necessary before he may be permitted to plead guilty or waive his right to counsel. In addition to determining that a defendant who seeks to plead guilty or waive counsel is competent, a trial court must satisfy itself that the waiver of his constitutional rights is knowing and voluntary. In this sense, there is a "heightened" standard for pleading guilty and for waiving the right to counsel, but it is not a heightened standard of competence.

This two-part inquiry is what we had in mind in *Westbrook*.[6] Thus, *Westbrook* stands only for the unremarkable proposition that when a defendant seeks to waive his right to counsel, a determination that he is competent to stand trial is not enough; the waiver must also be intelligent and voluntary before it can be accepted.

Requiring that a criminal defendant be competent has a modest aim: It seeks to ensure that he has the capacity to understand the proceedings and to assist counsel. While psychiatrists and scholars may find it useful to classify the various kinds and degrees of competence, and while States are free to adopt competency standards that are more elaborate than the *Dusky* formulation, the Due Process Clause does not impose these additional requirements.

Justice Kennedy, With Whom Justice Scalia Joins, Concurring in Part and Concurring in the Judgment

The Court compares the types of decisions made by one who goes to trial with the decisions required to plead guilty and waive the right to counsel. This comparison seems to suggest that there may have been a heightened standard of competency required by the Due Process Clause if the decisions were not equivalent. I have serious doubts about that proposition. In discussing the standard for a criminal defendant's competency to make decisions affecting his case, we should not confuse the content of the standard with the occasions for its application.

What is at issue here is whether the defendant has sufficient competence to take part in a criminal proceeding and to make the

---

[6] We do not mean to suggest, of course, that a court is required to make a competency determination in every case in which a defendant seeks to plead guilty or to waive his right to counsel. As in any criminal case, a competency determination is necessary only when a court has reason to doubt the defendant's competence.

decisions throughout its course. This is not to imply that mental competence is the only aspect of a defendant's state of mind that is relevant during criminal proceedings. Whether the defendant has made a knowing, intelligent, and voluntary decision to make certain fundamental choices during the course of criminal proceedings is another subject of judicial inquiry. That both questions might be implicated at any given point, however, does not mean that the inquiries cease to be discrete.

We have not suggested that the *Dusky* competency standard applies during the course of, but not before, trial. Instead, that standard is applicable from the time of arraignment through the return of a verdict. Although the *Dusky* standard refers to "ability to consult with a lawyer," the crucial component of the inquiry is the defendant's possession of "a reasonable degree of rational understanding." In other words, the focus of the *Dusky* formulation is on a particular level of mental functioning, which the ability

> **If a defendant elects to stand trial and to take the foolish course of acting as his own counsel, the law does not for that reason require any added degree of competence. (Kennedy, concurring)**

to consult counsel helps identify. The possibility that consultation will occur is not required for the standard to serve its purpose. If a defendant elects to stand trial and to take the foolish course of acting as his own counsel, the law does not for that reason require any added degree of competence.

The Due Process Clause does not mandate different standards of competency at various stages of or for different decisions made during the criminal proceedings. That was never the rule at common law, and it would take some extraordinary showing of the inadequacy of a single standard of competency for us to require States to employ heightened standards.

A single standard of competency to be applied throughout criminal proceedings does not offend any "principle of justice so rooted in the traditions and conscience of our people as to be ranked as fundamental" (*Medina v. California*). Nothing in our case law compels a contrary conclusion, and adoption of a rule setting out varying competency standards for each decision and stage of a criminal proceeding would disrupt the orderly course of trial and, from the standpoint of all parties, prove unworkable both at trial and on appellate review.

Justice Blackmun, With Whom
Justice Stevens Joins, Dissenting

The majority "rejects the notion that competence to plead guilty or to waive the right to counsel must be measured by a standard that is higher than (or even different from)" the standard for competence to stand trial articulated in *Dusky* and *Drope*. But the standard for competence to stand trial is specifically designed to measure a defendant's ability to "consult with counsel" and to "assist in preparing his defense." A finding that a defendant is competent to stand trial establishes only that he is capable of aiding his attorney in making the critical decisions required at trial or in plea negotiations. The reliability or even relevance of such a finding vanishes when its basic premise - that counsel will be present - ceases to exist. The question is no longer whether the defendant can proceed with an attorney, but whether he can proceed alone and uncounseled. I do not believe we place an excessive burden upon a trial court by requiring it to conduct a specific inquiry into that question at the juncture when a defendant whose competency already has been questioned seeks to waive counsel and represent himself.

The majority concludes that there is no need for such a hearing because a defendant who is found competent to stand trial with the assistance of counsel is, *ipso facto*,[7] competent to discharge counsel and represent himself. But the majority cannot isolate the term "competent" and apply it in a vacuum, divorced from its specific context. A person who is "competent" to play basketball is not thereby "competent" to play the violin. The majority's monolithic approach to competency is true to neither life nor the law. Competency for one purpose does not necessarily translate to competency for another purpose.

> **A person who is "competent" to play basketball is not thereby "competent" to play the violin. (Blackmun, dissenting)**

The majority asserts that "the competence that is required of a defendant seeking to waive his right to counsel is the competence to *waive the right*, not the competence to represent himself." But this assertion is simply incorrect. The majority's attempt to extricate the competence to waive the right to counsel from the competence to represent oneself is unavailing, because the former decision necessarily entails the latter. It is obvious that a defen-

---

[7] *ipso facto*. In and of itself.

dant who waives counsel must represent himself. Even Moran, who pleaded guilty, was required to defend himself during the penalty phase of the proceedings. And a defendant who is utterly incapable of conducting his own defense cannot be considered "competent" to make such a decision, any more than a person who chooses to leap out of a window in the belief that he can fly can be considered "competent" to make such a choice.

To try, convict, and punish one so helpless to defend himself contravenes fundamental principles of fairness and impugns the integrity of our criminal justice system. I cannot condone the decision to accept, without further inquiry, the self-destructive "choice" of a person who was so deeply medicated and who might well have been severely mentally ill. I dissent.

North Carolina v. Alford

400 U.S. 25 (1970)

Facts

Henry C. Alford was indicted on first-degree murder, a capital offense under North Carolina law. A defense attorney appointed to represent Alford questioned all but one of the witnesses the defendant said would substantiate his claim of innocence. The witnesses did not support Alford's story, however, but gave statements strongly indicating his guilt. Faced with strong evidence of guilt and no substantial evidentiary support for the claim of innocence, Alford's attorney recommended he plead guilty. The prosecution agreed to accept a plea of guilty to the lesser charge of second-degree murder. Before the plea was accepted by the trial court, a police officer's testimony summarized the facts of the state's case. Alford then took the stand and testified he had not committed the murder, but he was pleading guilty because he faced the death penalty if he did not do so. In response to questions from his attorney, he acknowledged having been informed of the difference between second- and first-degree murder and of his constitutional rights in the event he chose to go to trial. The guilty plea was ultimately accepted, and Alford was sentenced to 30-years imprisonment.

Procedural History

Alford sought post-conviction relief in state court raising the claim that his guilty plea was invalid because it was the product of fear and coercion. The state court denied relief, finding the plea to have been "willingly, knowingly, and understandingly" made on the advice of competent counsel and in the face of a strong prosecution case. Alford then petitioned for a writ of *habeas corpus*,[1] first in district court and then in the Court of Appeals for the Fourth Circuit. Both courts denied the writ. Two years later, Alford again petitioned for a writ of *habeas corpus* in district court, and it was also denied. On appeal, a divided panel of the Court of Appeals for the Fourth Circuit reversed on the ground

---

[1] writ of *habeas corpus*. A request to come before the court to ask for release from custody.

that Alford's guilty plea was made involuntarily. The U.S. Supreme Court granted *certiorari*.[2]

Issue

Is it constitutional error to accept a guilty plea from a defendant who denies guilt?

Holding

No. A guilty plea representing a voluntary and intelligent choice among alternatives available to a defendant, especially where the defendant is represented by competent counsel, is not compelled within the meaning of the Fifth Amendment merely because the plea is entered to avoid the possibility of the death penalty. Additionally, a defendant may voluntarily, knowingly, and understandingly consent to the imposition of a prison sentence even though he or she is unwilling to admit participation in the crime, or even if his guilty plea contains a protestation of innocence, when he intelligently concludes that his interests require a guilty plea and the record strongly indicates guilt.

Analysis

The standard for determining the validity of guilty pleas, the Supreme Court noted, is whether the plea represents a voluntary and intelligent choice among the alternative courses of action open to the defendant. That the defendant would not have pled guilty except for the opportunity to limit the possible penalty does not necessarily demonstrate that the guilty plea was not the product of a free and rational choice, especially where the defendant was represented by competent counsel whose advice was that the plea would be in the defendant's best interest.

Ordinarily, a judgment of conviction resting on a plea of guilty is justified by the defendant's admission he committed the crime and by his consent that judgment be entered without a trial of any kind. The plea usually subsumes both elements. State and lower federal courts have been divided upon whether a guilty plea can be accepted when it is accompanied by protestations of innocence and thus contains only a waiver of trial but no admission of guilt.

The Supreme Court noted that reasons other than guilt may induce a defendant to plead guilty, and defendants must be per-

---

[2] *certiorari*. A means of gaining appellate review.

mitted to make this decision for themselves. An individual accused of a crime may voluntarily, knowingly, and understandingly consent to the imposition of a prison sentence even if he is unwilling or unable to admit his participation in the acts constituting the crime. The Supreme Court said that its decision does not mean a trial judge must accept every constitutionally valid guilty plea merely because a defendant wishes to so plead. In the present case, however, the state had a strong case of first-degree murder against Alford, and confronted with the choice between a trial for first-degree murder and a plea of guilty to second-degree murder, Alford's choice was considered quite reasonable.

Edited Excerpts[3]

North Carolina v. Henry C. Alford

Supreme Court of the United States

Appeal from order of the United States District Court
for the Middle District of North Carolina, at Greensboro

400 U.S. 25

November 23, 1970

White, J., delivered the opinion of the Court, in which Burger, C. J., and Harlan, Stewart, and Blackmun, J., joined. Black, J., filed a statement concurring in the judgment. Brennan, J., filed a dissenting opinion, in which Douglas and Marshall, J., joined.

On December 2, 1963, Alford was indicted for first-degree murder, a capital offense under North Carolina law. The court appointed an attorney to represent him, and this attorney questioned all but one of the various witnesses who appellee said would substantiate his claim of innocence. The witnesses, however, did not support Alford's story but gave statements that strongly indicated his guilt. Faced with strong evidence of guilt and no substantial evidentiary support for the claim of innocence, Alford's attorney recommended that he plead guilty, but left the ultimate decision to Alford himself. The prosecutor agreed to ac-

---

[3] Readers are advised to quote only from the original published cases. See pages vii-viii.

cept a plea of guilty to a charge of second-degree murder, and on December 10, 1963, Alford pleaded guilty to the reduced charge.

Before the plea was finally accepted by the trial court, the court heard the sworn testimony of a police officer who summarized the State's case. Two other witnesses besides Alford were also heard. Although there was no eyewitness to the crime, the testimony indicated that shortly before the killing Alford took his gun from his house, stated his intention to kill the victim, and returned home with the declaration that he had carried out the killing. After the summary presentation of the State's case, Alford took the stand and testified that he had not committed the murder but that he was pleading guilty because he faced the threat of the death penalty if he did not do so.[4] In response to the questions of his counsel, he acknowledged that his counsel had informed him of the difference between second- and first-degree murder and of his rights in case he chose to go to trial.[5] The trial court then asked appellee if, in light of his denial of guilt, he still desired to plead guilty to second-degree murder and appellee answered, "Yes, sir. I plead guilty on - from the circumstances that he [Alford's attorney] told me." After eliciting information about Alford's prior criminal record, which was a long one, the trial court sentenced him to 30 years imprisonment, the maximum penalty for second-degree murder.

Alford sought post-conviction relief in the state court. Among the claims raised was the claim that his plea of guilty was invalid because it was the product of fear and coercion. After a hearing, the state court in 1965 found that the plea was "willingly, knowingly, and

> **"I'm not guilty but I plead guilty."**

---

[4] After giving his version of the events of the night of the murder, Alford stated: "I pleaded guilty on second degree murder because they said there is too much evidence, but I ain't shot no man, but I take the fault for the other man. We never had an argument in our life and I just pleaded guilty because they said if I didn't they would gas me for it, and that is all." In response to questions from his attorney, Alford affirmed that he had consulted several times with his attorney and with members of his family and had been informed of his rights if he chose to plead not guilty. Alford then reaffirmed his decision to plead guilty to second-degree murder: "Q. [by Alford's attorney]. And you authorized me to tender a plea of guilty to second degree murder before the court?" "A. Yes, sir." "Q. And in doing that, that you have again affirmed your decision on that point?" "A. Well, I'm still pleading that you all got me to plead guilty. I plead the other way, circumstantial evidence; that the jury will prosecute me on - on the second. You told me to plead guilty, right. I don't - I'm not guilty but I plead guilty."

[5] At the state court hearing on post-conviction relief, the testimony confirmed that Alford had been fully informed by his attorney as to his rights on a plea of not guilty and as to the consequences of a plea of guilty.

understandingly" made on the advice of competent counsel and in the face of a strong prosecution case. Subsequently, Alford petitioned for a writ of *habeas corpus*, first in the United States District Court for the Middle District of North Carolina, and then in the Court of Appeals for the Fourth Circuit. Both courts denied the writ on the basis of the state court's findings that Alford voluntarily and knowingly agreed to plead guilty. In 1967, Alford again petitioned for a writ of *habeas corpus* in the District Court for the Middle District of North Carolina. That court, without an evidentiary hearing, again denied relief on the grounds that the guilty plea was voluntary and waived all defenses and nonjurisdictional defects in any prior stage of the proceedings, and that the findings of the state court in 1965 clearly required rejection of Alford's claim that he was denied effective assistance of counsel prior to pleading guilty. On appeal, a divided panel of the Court of Appeals for the Fourth Circuit reversed on the ground that Alford's guilty plea was made involuntarily. In reaching its conclusion, the Court of Appeals relied heavily on *United States v. Jackson*, which the court read to require invalidation of the North Carolina statutory framework for the imposition of the death penalty because North Carolina statutes encouraged defendants to waive constitutional rights by the promise of no more than life imprisonment if a guilty plea was offered and accepted. Conceding that [*United States v. Jackson*] did not require the automatic invalidation of pleas of guilty entered under the North Carolina statutes, the Court of Appeals ruled that Alford's guilty plea was involuntary because its principal motivation was fear of the death penalty. By this standard, even if both the judge and the jury had possessed the power to impose the death penalty for first-degree murder or if guilty pleas to capital charges had not been permitted, Alford's plea of guilty to second-degree murder should still have been rejected because [it was] impermissibly induced by his desire to eliminate the possibility of a death sentence. We vacate the judgment of the Court of Appeals and remand the case for further proceedings.

We held in *Brady v. United States*, that a plea of guilty which would not have been entered except for the defendant's desire to avoid a possible death penalty and to limit the maximum penalty to life imprisonment or a term of years

> **The standard was and remains whether the plea represents a voluntary and intelligent choice among the alternative courses of action open to the defendant.**

was not for that reason compelled within the meaning of the Fifth

Amendment. *United States v. Jackson* established no new test for determining the validity of guilty pleas. The standard was and remains whether the plea represents a voluntary and intelligent choice among the alternative courses of action open to the defendant. That he would not have pleaded except for the opportunity to limit the possible penalty does not necessarily demonstrate that the plea of guilty was not the product of a free and rational choice, especially where the defendant was represented by competent counsel whose advice was that the plea would be to the defendant's advantage. The standard fashioned and applied by the Court of Appeals was therefore erroneous and we would, without more, vacate and remand the case for further proceedings.

As previously recounted, after Alford's plea of guilty was offered and the State's case was placed before the judge, Alford denied that he had committed the murder but reaffirmed his desire to plead guilty to avoid a possible death sentence and to limit the penalty to the 30-year maximum provided for second-degree murder. Ordinarily, a judgment of conviction resting on a plea of guilty is justified by the defendant's admission that he committed the crime charged against him and his consent that judgment be entered without a trial of any kind. The plea usually subsumes both elements, and justifiably so, even though there is no separate, express admission by the defendant that he committed the particular acts claimed to constitute the crime charged in the indictment. Here Alford entered his plea but accompanied it with the statement that he had not shot the victim. If Alford's statements were to be credited as sincere assertions of his innocence, there obviously existed a factual and legal dispute between him and the State. Without more, it might be argued that the conviction entered on his guilty plea was invalid, since his assertion of innocence [negated] any admission of guilt.

In addition to Alford's statement, however, the court had heard an account of the events on the night of the murder, including information from Alford's acquaintances that he had departed from his home with his gun stating his intention to kill and that he had later declared that he had carried out his intention. Nor had Alford wavered in his desire to have the trial court determine his guilt without a jury trial. Although denying the charge against him, he nevertheless preferred the dispute between him and the State to be settled by the judge in the context of a guilty plea proceeding rather than by a formal trial. Thereupon, with the State's telling evidence and Alford's denial before it, the trial court proceeded to convict and sentence Alford for second-degree murder.

State and lower federal courts are divided upon whether a guilty plea can be accepted when it is accompanied by protestations of innocence and hence contains only a waiver of trial but no admission of guilt. Some courts, giving expression to the principle that "our law only authorizes a conviction where guilt is shown," require that trial judges reject such pleas. But others have concluded that they should not "force any defense on a defendant in a criminal case," particularly when advancement of the defense might "end in disaster." They have argued that, since "guilt, or the degree of guilt, is at times uncertain and elusive," "an accused, though believing in or entertaining doubts respecting his innocence, might reasonably conclude a jury would be convinced of his guilt and that he would fare better in the sentence by pleading guilty." As one state court observed nearly a century ago, "reasons other than the fact that he is guilty may induce a defendant to so plead, and he must be permitted to judge for himself in this respect."

This Court has not confronted this precise issue, but prior decisions do yield relevant principles. In *Lynch v. Overholser*, Lynch, who had been charged in the Municipal Court of the District of Columbia with drawing and negotiating bad checks, a misdemeanor punishable by a maximum of one year in jail, sought to enter a plea of guilty, but the trial judge refused to accept the plea since a psychiatric report in the judge's possession indicated that Lynch had been suffering from "a

> *Reasons other than the fact that he is guilty may induce a defendant to so plead, and he must be permitted to judge for himself in this respect.*

manic depressive psychosis, at the time of the crime charged," and hence might have been not guilty by reason of insanity. The Court expressly refused to rule that Lynch had an absolute right to have his guilty plea accepted, but implied that there would have been no constitutional error had his plea been accepted even though evidence before the judge indicated that there was a valid defense.

Thus, while most pleas of guilty consist of both a waiver of trial and an express admission of guilt, the latter element is not a constitutional requisite to the imposition of a criminal penalty. An individual accused of a crime may voluntarily, knowingly, and understandingly consent to the imposition of a prison sentence even if he is unwilling or unable to admit his participation in the acts constituting the crime.

Nor can we perceive any material difference between a plea that refuses to admit commission of the criminal act and a plea containing a protestation of innocence when, as in the instant case, a defendant intelligently concludes that his interests require entry of a guilty plea and the record before the judge contains strong evidence of actual guilt. Here the State had a strong case of first-degree murder against Alford. Whether he realized or disbelieved his guilt, he insisted on his plea because in his view he had absolutely nothing to gain by a trial and much to gain by pleading. Because of the overwhelming evidence against him, a trial was precisely what neither Alford nor his attorney desired. Confronted with the choice between a trial for first-degree murder, on the one hand, and a plea of guilty to second-degree murder, on the other, Alford quite reasonably chose the latter and thereby limited the maximum penalty to a 30-year term. When his plea is viewed in light of the evidence against him, which substantially negated his claim of innocence and which further provided a means by which the judge could test whether the plea was being intelligently entered, its validity cannot be seriously questioned. In view of the strong factual basis for the plea demonstrated by the State and Alford's clearly expressed desire to enter it despite his professed belief in his innocence, we hold that the trial judge did not commit constitutional error in accepting it.[6]

> **Because of the overwhelming evidence against him, a trial was precisely what neither Alford nor his attorney desired.**

Relying on *United States v. Jackson*, Alford now argues in effect that the State should not have allowed him this choice but should have insisted on proving him guilty of murder in the first degree. The States in their wisdom may take this course by statute or otherwise and may prohibit the practice of accepting pleas to lesser included offenses under any circumstances. But this is not the mandate of the Fourteenth Amendment[7] and the Bill of Rights. The prohibitions against involuntary or unintelligent pleas should not be relaxed, but neither should an exercise in arid logic render those constitutional guarantees counterproductive and put in jeopardy the very human values they were meant to preserve. The Court of Appeals for the Fourth Circuit was in error

---

[6] Our holding does not mean that a trial judge must accept every constitutionally valid guilty plea merely because a defendant wishes so to plead. A criminal defendant does not have an absolute right under the Constitution to have his guilty plea accepted by the court, although the States may by statute or otherwise confer such a right. Likewise, the States may bar their courts from accepting guilty pleas from any defendants who assert their innocence.

[7] Fourteenth Amendment (Section 1). See Appendix B (p. 262).

to find Alford's plea of guilty invalid because it was made to avoid the possibility of the death penalty. That court's judgment directing the issuance of the writ of *habeas corpus* is vacated and the case is remanded to the Court of Appeals for further proceedings consistent with this opinion.

It is so ordered.

Mr. Justice Brennan, With Whom Mr. Justice Douglas and Mr. Justice Marshall Join, Dissenting

Last Term, this Court held, over my dissent, that a plea of guilty may validly be induced by an unconstitutional threat to subject the defendant to the risk of death, so long as the plea is entered in open court and the defendant is represented by competent counsel who is aware of the threat, albeit not of its unconstitutionality. Today the Court makes clear that its previous holding was intended to

> **Alford was "so gripped by fear of the death penalty" that his decision to plead guilty was not voluntary. (Brennan, dissenting)**

apply even when the record demonstrates that the actual effect of the unconstitutional threat was to induce a guilty plea from a defendant who was unwilling to admit his guilt. I adhere to the view that, in any given case, the influence of such an unconstitutional threat "must necessarily be given weight in determining the voluntariness of a plea." And, without reaching the question whether due process permits the entry of judgment upon a plea of guilty accompanied by a contemporaneous denial of acts constituting the crime, I believe that at the very least such a denial of guilt is also a relevant factor in determining whether the plea was voluntarily and intelligently made. With these factors in mind, it is sufficient in my view to state that the facts set out in the majority opinion demonstrate that Alford was "so gripped by fear of the death penalty" that his decision to plead guilty was not voluntary but was "the product of duress as much so as choice reflecting physical constraint." Accordingly, I would affirm the judgment of the Court of Appeals.

United States v. Greer

158 F.3d 228 (1998)

Facts

Charles Randell Greer was convicted of kidnapping and related charges. It was the conclusion of the trial court, based on its
own observations and the opinions of mental health experts, that
Greer had feigned mental impairment. The government moved
that the proposed sentencing range be increased for obstruction of
justice because of the malingering. The trial judge agreed. Greer's
sentence was increased by 25 months. Greer appealed to the
Court of Appeals for the Fifth Circuit.

Issue

Does malingering constitute obstruction of justice under the
U.S. Sentencing Guidelines?

Holding

Yes. Malingering, determined by a preponderance of the evidence standard, constitutes obstruction of justice and can be punished by a sentence enhancement.

Analysis

The Fifth Circuit concluded malingering was analogous to the
class of conduct that warrants a sentence enhancement. The conduct required a significant amount of planning and presented an
inherently high risk that justice would be obstructed. It was different than behavior that reflected a spur of the moment decision
or which stemmed from mere panic.

Edited Excerpts[1]

United States of America, Plaintiff-Appellee, v. Charles Randell Greer, Defendant-Appellant

In the United States Court of Appeals for the Fifth Circuit

158 F.3d 228

October 16, 1998

Before King, Smith, and Parker, Circuit Judges

King, Circuit Judge

Defendant-Appellant Charles Randell Greer appeals the district court's enhancement of his sentence for obstruction of justice. We affirm.

During the summer of 1994, defendant-appellee Charles Randell Greer, a convicted felon with a lengthy criminal record, one previous determination of incompetency, and numerous commitments to psychiatric facilities, was homeless. Joyce Cantrell, a resident of Lubbock, Texas for whom Greer had done odd jobs, offered to let him stay in her garage apartment, and he moved in on July 16, 1994. That evening, he asked to use the telephone in Cantrell's house. Cantrell allowed him to do so, but when he finished his conversation, he was distraught and, without permission, entered her bedroom and lay down on her bed. When Cantrell asked him to leave, he grabbed her wrists and told her, "Don't cause me any problems." In order to appease Greer, Cantrell offered to cook him dinner, and when he returned to the bedroom, she escaped from the house and called the police. Greer had left by the time the police arrived, but when Cantrell returned the next morning, she discovered human excrement smeared in the bathroom and bedroom, and a .22 caliber revolver was missing.

The evidence at trial showed that after Cantrell left her house on the evening of July 16, Greer went to the home of Arthur Follows, another Lubbock resident for whom he had done odd jobs. Follows had befriended Greer in the past, giving him a ride to the hospital when Greer claimed that his grandfather had attempted

---

[1] Readers are advised to quote only from the original published cases. See pages vii-viii.

suicide and then to Greer's uncle's house when Greer decided that he would rather see the uncle. At about 10:00 or 11:00 p.m., an agitated Greer arrived at Follows' home and asked to take a shower. Follows permitted him to do so, but told him that he would have to leave afterward. After Greer showered, however, he went to Follows' bedroom. Normally soft-spoken and shy, he began cursing loudly, telling Follows that no one cared about him.

At that point, Follows ordered Greer to leave. Greer then struck Follows, who fell back onto the bed, and bound him at gunpoint. He told Follows that he wanted Follows to drive him away from Lubbock because he wanted to kill himself, and the two men left in Follows' car. Greer, who kept the gun pointed at Follows with his finger

> *"Now, you better take these thoughts into consideration, get with the program, and stop acting like a fool."*

on the trigger, told Follows to drive him to Clovis, New Mexico. During the journey, Greer drank heavily and continued to complain that no one cared about him. When Follows reached Clovis, he began to pull into the bus station, enraging Greer, who jammed the revolver into Follows' ear and then his side. Greer ordered Follows to drive to Albuquerque, but when they arrived, Greer became very sad, apologized to Follows, and asked to be taken to a motel, where he paid for a room with Follows' Master-Card. He indicated that he had achieved the purpose of the kidnapping - to be a long way from his family and friends when he committed suicide - and apologized again. He then allowed Follows to leave and entered the motel room alone. Follows immediately called the police, who arrested Greer at the motel.

The post-arrest events were even stranger than the kidnapping itself. After Greer's arrest, a doctor attached to the Bernalillo County Detention Center in New Mexico gave him a prescription for Thorazine and Elavil. Greer was also found incompetent to stand trial on the New Mexico state charges stemming from Follows' kidnapping. On November 14, 1994, pursuant to a joint motion filed by Greer and the Government, the district court ordered Greer committed to the custody of the Attorney General to undergo a competency evaluation. After a 1½ month evaluation at the United States Medical Center for Federal Prisoners in Springfield, Missouri, Greer returned to Lubbock. The district court held a competency hearing on April 21, 1995. After local jail personnel and the FBI case agent testified to evidence tending to demonstrate Greer's competency, the Government called Dr. Richard Frederick, Greer's forensic psychologist at Springfield, who testified not only that Greer was competent to stand trial, but that he was feigning psychotic illness. Dr. Frederick stated that he came to his conclusion based, in part, on a three-page narrative Greer wrote that cogently set forth his "understanding" of the crime - namely, that Follows had sexually assaulted him and had concocted the kidnapping story to save himself from punishment. Greer called only one witness, a local psychiatrist named Preston Shaw, who testified that Greer was incompetent. The district court determined that Greer was competent.

As trial preparation continued, Greer's bizarre behavior prompted his attorney to file another motion to determine competency. The district court initially denied the request but later granted it after the Government declined to oppose the motion. Greer was examined by Dr. Ross Taylor, a psychiatrist with the Texas Department of Corrections. Taylor determined that Greer was incompetent, the Government acquiesced to allowing Greer to be adjudicated incompetent, and on February 8, 1996, the district court executed an agreed order committing Greer to the custody of the Attorney General until such time as his competency was restored.

On June 25, 1996, after receiving a psychiatric evaluation from the Federal Medical Center in Rochester, Minnesota, the district court ordered a second competency hearing. On July 17, 1996, the court convened a competency hearing at which Dr. Mary Alice Conroy, a psychologist who had evaluated Greer during his commitment at Rochester, testified. Conroy stated that because Greer was

> **The Government objected to Greer's pre-sentence report because it did not enhance his sentence for obstructing justice.**

referred for restoration of competence, the medical staff initially presumed that he suffered from a serious mental disease that rendered him incompetent. But after observing Greer for nearly two months, Greer's treating psychiatrist, Dr. Sigerson, was unable to find any active psychotic process or serious mental disease. During Greer's case conference, in which six members of the medical staff involved in Greer's treatment and evaluation, including Dr. Sigerson and Dr. Conroy, participated, it was concluded that there was no evidence of psychotic process. Conroy opined that Greer was a malingerer, although she conceded that Greer had a personality disorder with antisocial and borderline tendencies that could not be treated. The day before trial, the district court found not only that Greer was competent but that he had feigned mental illness.

Greer's trial began on August 7, 1996. At approximately 10:30 a.m. on the first day, after *voir dire*[2] and while the attorneys were making peremptory challenges, the marshals informed the district court that Greer had taken his clothes off and attempted to flush them down the holding cell toilet. During the resulting delay, Greer spit up between ten and sixteen half-dollar-sized splotches of blood and was taken to a local hospital. In Greer's absence, at approximately 11:15 a.m., the court called the names of the twelve jurors, seated them, administered their oath, and recessed the trial until 1:30 p.m.

The prosecution then called the jail's director of infirmary services, Lauren McQuitty, to testify. McQuitty stated that an evaluation of Greer at the hospital had determined a mucosal abrasion in his mouth to be the cause of the bleeding; that such abrasions commonly were caused by self-inflicted scratches; and that Greer's fingernails were about an inch long. McQuitty also noted that, from the appearance of the blood, it appeared that Greer was gagging himself, rather than vomiting blood from the stomach,

> **Greer received a 210-month sentence with the obstruction of justice enhancement, whereas without the enhancement the maximum sentence he could have received was 185 months.**

intestine, or liver. After McQuitty's testimony, the court stated the following on the record, but outside the presence of the jury: "I am finding based upon the medical report that the defendant created an abrasion in his mouth, so as to cause some bleeding, which in my mind is a further deliberate attempt on his part - I am talking about Mr. Greer - to derail the trial of this case. Now, Mr. Greer, before I bring the jury back in, I want you to listen to me very carefully. I think you are a malingerer. I have found you competent to stand trial. We are going to have this trial. If you act up or try to disrupt this trial while you are in this courtroom, I am going to have you removed from this courtroom, and we will try the case in your absence. Mr. Greer, I have told you this once before, but you had better get very serious about defending this case. Now, you better take these thoughts into consideration, get with the program, and stop acting like a fool." Greer responded, "Yes, sir, your honor." Toward the end of the day, during the testimony of an Albuquerque, New Mexico police officer, Greer suddenly jumped out of his chair and shouted, "Get it away. Stop." Greer yelled "Stop!" once more before he was subdued. Outside

---

[2] *voir dire.* An examination of prospective jurors.

the presence of the jury, the court ordered Greer removed from the courtroom, and the proceedings continued without Greer for the remainder of the first day. The jury convicted Greer in his absence of all the counts against him.

At sentencing, the Government objected to Greer's pre-sentence report because it did not enhance his sentence for obstructing justice. The Government argued that because Greer had feigned mental illness prior to and during (by flushing his clothes in the toilet, scratching his throat to give the appearance of throwing up blood, and shouting and jumping out of his chair) trial, the court should increase his offense level pursuant to [Federal] Sentencing Guidelines. The district court granted the Government's objection, resulting in a two-level offense level enhancement for obstruction of justice. The court stated at sentencing: "I will add two points for obstruction of justice. I find that the Defendant is a malingerer, that he feigned a mental illness, thereby causing the Court and the Bureau of Prisons to waste a considerable amount of time and effort in addressing that particular situation." Greer thus received a 210-month sentence with the obstruction of justice enhancement, whereas without the enhancement the maximum sentence he could have received was 185 months. Greer appealed.

We must determine whether a defendant's feigning incompetence is the type of conduct to which [the guidelines] apply. If it is not, then we must reverse as a matter of law and remand for resentencing. If it is, we must consider whether the district court properly applied [the guidelines] in this case.

We begin our analysis by examining the Guidelines themselves [which are] titled "Obstructing or Impeding the Administration of Justice" and read: "If the defendant willfully obstructed or impeded, or attempted to obstruct or impede, the administration of justice during the investigation, prosecution, or sentencing of the instant offense, increase the offense level by 2 levels." The Guidelines

> **Malingering is more like the types of conduct to which the sentencing guidelines apply than those to which it does not.**

Manual does not define "obstruct," but the application notes provide some guidance as to the type of conduct to which the obstruction enhancement applies. For example, although "obstructive conduct can vary widely in nature, degree of planning, and seriousness," [the guidelines are] not intended to punish a defendant for the exercise of a constitutional right. The application notes also list examples of the type of conduct to which the obstruction enhancement applies: (1) threatening, intimidating, or otherwise unlawfully influencing a co-defendant, witness, or juror, directly or indirectly, or attempting to do so; (2) committing, suborning, or attempting to suborn perjury; (3) producing or attempting to produce a false, altered, or counterfeit document or record during an official investigation or judicial proceeding; (4) destroying or concealing or directing or procuring another person to destroy or conceal evidence that is material to an official investigation or judicial proceeding, or attempting to do so; (5) escaping or attempting to escape from custody before trial or sentencing; or willfully failing to appear, as ordered, for a judicial proceeding; (6) providing materially false information to a judge or magistrate; (7) providing materially false information to a probation officer in respect to a pre-sentence or other investigation for the court; and (8) other conduct prohibited by [statute].

The application notes also provide a nonexhaustive list of the types of conduct to which the guideline does not apply, but which may be punished with a greater sentence within the otherwise applicable guideline range: (1) providing a false name or identification document at arrest, except where such conduct actually resulted in a significant hindrance to the investigation or prosecution of the instant offense; (2) making false statements, not under oath, to law enforcement officers, unless it is a materially false statement that significantly obstructed or impeded the official investigation or prosecution of the instant offense; (3) providing incomplete or misleading information, not amounting to a material falsehood, in respect to a pre-sentence investigation; and (4) avoiding or fleeing from arrest.

Thus, the commentary does not explicitly refer to the act of feigning incompetence in order to avoid trial, conviction, or sentencing. Our analysis of the application notes convinces us, however, that such malingering is more like the types of conduct to which [the guidelines] apply than those to which it does not. In general, the acts in the latter category, while dishonest, carry little risk of significantly impeding the investigation or prosecution of a case and require substantially less planning than those in the category of behavior to which [the guidelines apply]. For example, providing a false name at arrest and making false, unsworn statements to law enforcement officers trigger [the guidelines] only if they actually significantly obstruct or impede the investigation or prosecution. Simi-

> *Putting on the pretense of incompetency demands not only dramatic ability but planning and resolve.*

larly, providing incomplete or misleading information in respect
to a probation officer runs afoul of [the guidelines] only if the
falsehoods are material. Furthermore, it may be that unsworn
communications to law enforcement officers, not to mention decisions to flee from arrest, are likely to be made on the spur of the
moment and reflect panic, confusion, or mistake rather than a
deliberate attempt to obstruct justice. In short, [the guidelines
exclude] conduct that does not tend to reflect a considered effort
to derail investigations and prosecutions or significantly increase
the risk that this in fact will happen.

The types of conduct listed are quite different. They involve
egregiously wrongful behavior whose execution requires a significant amount of planning and presents an inherently high risk
that justice will in fact be obstructed. Putting on the pretense of
incompetency demands not only dramatic ability but planning
and resolve. Unlike providing false identification at arrest and
avoiding arrest altogether, it is not the result of a spur of the
moment decision. Nor can it stem from merely panic, confusion,
or mistake. And, of course, a criminal defendant's sanity is always
material: If he succeeds at convincing the court of his incompetency, he does not only increase his chances of acquittal, as he
would if he committed perjury or falsified a record; he makes it
impossible even to try him. Thus, it appears, from an analysis of
the text of the Guidelines Manual alone, that [the guidelines ap-
ply] to the act of feigning incompetency.

Although there are no cases precisely on point, the courts
have found behavior similar in purpose or effect to feigning incompetency to trigger [the guidelines]. For example, a court may
use the obstruction enhancement to punish a defendant who lies
on the stand about his mental state (*United States v. Abdelkoui*;
affirming the district court's application of [the guidelines] where
the defendant claimed that he was incapacitated by attacks of
hypoglycemia that prevented him from forming the requisite intent and was later determined to be lying). [The guidelines also
apply] to material lies about physical condition and its effect on
mental state (*United States v. Hall*; approving [an] enhancement
where the defendant falsely claimed that his confession could not
be voluntary because it was the product of a methamphetamine-
induced psychosis). In the same vein, providing false handwriting
samples may also trigger the enhancement (*United States v. Yusufu*; affirming [an] enhancement for a defendant who willfully
disguised a handwriting exemplar to be provided to the FBI for
comparison to writings that were to be introduced at trial; *United
States v. Valdez*; upholding an obstruction of justice adjustment

based in part on the defendant's ultimately unsuccessful attempt to disguise his handwriting when giving exemplars under subpoena for comparison with his date book of drug records). Failing to report to give samples is also an obstruction of justice. For example, the Ninth Circuit has held that a defendant claiming diminished capacity who refuses to submit to court-ordered psychiatric testing so that the prosecution can respond to his defense obstructs justice within the meaning of [the guidelines] (*United States v. Fontenot*). Defendants who refuse to provide court-ordered handwriting samples have also been found to obstruct justice (*United States v. Taylor; United States v. Ruth*). A defendant who feigns incompetency essentially provides a false "sample" lying about his psychiatric condition in order to convince the court that he cannot be found guilty - for that matter, even put on trial.

The fact that each of the above examples, unlike feigning incompetency, fits under one of the categories of behavior that triggers the obstruction enhancement is a distinction without a difference. The application note [in the guidelines] makes clear that its list is nonexhaustive, and as the Seventh Circuit has noted, the guideline is concerned more with the effect of potentially obstructive conduct than with formalistic definitions (*United States v. Harrison*; "Unquestionably, the guideline is less concerned with whether the false information was given under oath than with the information's effect on a judicial decision or investigation"). Moreover, feigning incompetence may well fall under a broad interpretation of producing or attempting to produce a false record: A defendant who playacts psychosis essentially tries to create a record that includes inaccurate testimony and factual conclusions. For example, a defendant violates [statute] when he tells a potential witness a false story as if the story were true, intending that the witness believe the story and repeat it to a grand jury (*United States v. Rodolitz United States v. Gabriel; United States v. Bordallo*).

> *A defendant who playacts psychosis essentially tries to create a record that includes inaccurate testimony and factual conclusions.*

Similarly, a defendant who feigns incompetency misrepresents his psychiatric condition to his examiners, intending that they will believe him and convey their inaccurate impressions to the court.

Greer contended at oral argument that [the guidelines apply] only when the underlying conduct constitutes a crime in and of itself. Because it is not a crime to move the court for a competency hearing or to jump up and cry out in court, he claims, his behavior lies outside the scope of the enhancement. Our review of the record reveals, however, that the district court found that Greer obstructed justice not because he requested a competency hearing and disrupted his trial, but because he feigned incompetency.

Greer's second argument, that applying enhancements to defendants who feign incompetency impermissibly chills their constitutional right not to be tried if they are incompetent, has somewhat more merit. It is well-established that [the guidelines] cannot be applied to punish a defendant for the exercise of a constitutional right. It is equally well-established that the Due Process Clause of the Fourteenth Amendment[3] prohibits the criminal prosecution of a defendant who is not competent to stand trial (*Drope; Pate*). Thus, [the guidelines] cannot be used to enhance the sentence of a defendant simply because he or his attorney requests competency hearings.

The Supreme Court confronted an analogous problem in *United States v. Dunnigan*, in which the Supreme Court upheld the application of the obstruction enhancement to a defendant who committed perjury at trial, despite her argument that [doing so] would chill her constitutional right to testify on her own behalf. In rejecting this argument, the Court pointed out that "our authorities do not impose a categorical ban on every governmental action affecting the strategic decisions of an accused, including decisions whether or not to exercise constitutional rights." The Court further observed that "a defendant's right to testify does not include a right to commit perjury." Moreover, the Court found, enhancements for perjury do not create an unconstitutionally high risk that district courts will order enhancement as a matter of course whenever the accused takes the stand and is found guilty, because if the defendant challenges a sentence increase based on perjured testimony, the trial court must make findings to support all the elements of a perjury violation in the specific case.

Similarly, applying the obstruction enhancement to defendants who willfully feign incompetence in order to avoid trial and punishment does not unconstitutionally chill defendant's right to seek a competency hearing. While a criminal defendant possesses a constitutional right to a competency hearing if a *bona fide* doubt exists as to his competency, he surely does not have the right to create a doubt as to his competency or to increase the chances that he will be found incompetent by feigning mental illness. Of

---

[3] Due Process Clause of the Fourteenth Amendment (Section 1). See Appendix B (p. 262).

course, our finding that [the guidelines] may be applied to malingerers is not meant to encourage or justify automatically increasing sentences for all defendants who seek a competency hearing and ultimately are found competent. As in *Dunnigan*, if a defendant challenges a sentence increase based on feigned incompetency, the district court must make findings to support its ruling. Nor does our decision today put defense counsel to the Hobson's choice of forgoing competency hearings for a client who may well be incompetent (and thereby creating grounds for an ineffective assistance of counsel claim) or requesting such hearings and exposing the client to the risk of [an] enhancement if he is ultimately found competent. Counsel should warn his client that feigning incompetency, whether to create doubt as to his competency so as to prod his attorney into requesting competency hearings or to convince the court that he cannot stand trial, will trigger [an] enhancement. If the defendant is found competent, and the court later determines that he feigned incompetence in order to delay or avoid his day of reckoning, it will apply the enhancement. If the court finds, however, that the defendant did not feign incompetence but that there was simply a *bona fide* doubt about his mental health that did not rise to the level of incompetence, then it may not increase the sentence. In either case, the defendant and his attorney need not choose between a competency hearing and avoiding an obstruction enhancement.

[E]ven if there is sufficient evidence to justify a competency hearing absent the defendant's machinations, feigning incompetency during a psychiatric evaluation would seem always to increase the risk that the defendant will erroneously be found incompetent. More important, [the guideline] itself indicates that it applies to attempts to obstruct justice as well as to the actual obstruction of justice. Even if the defendant's actions could have had no impact whatsoever on the course of events leading to his being found competent, his attempt to manipulate the judicial system reflects on his character and is therefore a relevant consideration at sentencing.

> **A criminal defendant does not have the right to create a doubt as to his competency or to increase the chances that he will be found incompetent by feigning mental illness.**

Finally, we must determine whether, because a defendant's diagnosed personality disorders complicate the task of determining whether his obstructive acts were "willful," the Government must show willfulness by a higher standard of proof than mere preponderance of the evidence. In support of this evidentiary standard, Greer points out that the Supreme Court has observed that it is still an open question whether "some heightened standard of proof might apply to sentencing determinations which bear significantly on the severity of sentence," *Almendarez-Torres v. United States*, and that in the analogous situation of insanity issues, Congress requires courts to use the "clear and convincing" standard when making particular determinations. We can see no reason to deviate from the standard used in all other aspects of the sentencing process.

We therefore review the district court's conclusion that Greer obstructed justice for clear error, keeping in mind that the Government need show, and the court need find, only by a preponderance of the evidence that Greer feigned incompetence in order to delay or avoid his trial. The district court did not clearly err. The Government's expert testified that although Greer suffered from antisocial and borderline personality disorders, he was capable of controlling his behavior. A quantity of other evidence supports the court's finding of willful malingering. For instance, Greer made false statements that he did not know his attorney; did not know what he was charged with; could not recite the alphabet; and could not tell what year it was. When told that his urinating out the slot of his cell door would fail to convince his doctors that he was incompetent and that successful malingering required that he urinate or defecate in his cell, he ceased urinating out the slot and began defecating in a corner of his cell. While he often conversed with nonmedical personnel, he refused to speak to his doctors and tried to avoid being placed in housing where he could be observed easily. Although he claimed to benefit from antipsychotic drugs, his behavior did not change when he stopped taking them. Finally, Dr. Richard Frederick of the Federal Medical Center at Springfield, Missouri administered a Forced Choice Test to Greer, whose pattern of responses suggested that he was feigning [cognitive impairment].

The law, of course, requires not only that the defendant commit affirmative acts that tend to create an appearance of incompetency, but that he do so with the specific intent of obstructing justice. In this case, we have only circumstantial evidence of Greer's intent. We do not believe, however, that the Government must produce proof as direct and incontrovertible as, say, a tape recording of the defendant confessing his plan to feign incompetency in order to delay or avoid trial and punishment. On the other hand, we recognize that a determination by the district court, after a competency hearing, that a defendant is competent to stand trial often will entail a conclusion that the defendant's alleged mental illness is at least partially feigned, and we do not suggest that every instance of feigned mental illness justifies an enhancement for obstruction of justice. The district court may find from circumstantial evidence that the defendant engaged in a conscious and deliberate attempt to obstruct or impede the administration of justice. In this case, there was evidence that Greer engaged in a sustained pattern of appearing considerably more impaired than he was, and when he was told that certain actions would not convince the experts that he was in fact insane, he modified his behavior. The district court did not clearly err in finding that Greer willfully feigned mental illness in a conscious and deliberate effort to delay, and perhaps avoid altogether, his day of reckoning on the grave offenses with which he was charged.

For the foregoing reasons, we affirm Greer's sentence.

Implications for Examiners

Different terminology sometimes creates confusion between the court and mental health examiners. *McDonald* makes it clear that clinicians must recognize and respect the differences in language and strive to translate mental health concepts into language the court finds useful. *Medina* and *Cooper* underscore the importance of providing courts with evidence they can balance to make a decision about competency. Evidence is preferred to conclusory pronouncements by the clinician. As *Medina* and *Cooper* show, an individual can be competent in one jurisdiction, but not in another. Competency is ultimately a legal "condition," reflecting the prevailing values of statutory and case law at a particular time in a particular jurisdiction. The Supreme Court's finding in *Cooper* makes it less likely that jurisdictions will differ substantively on what constitutes incompetency, given that most jurisdictions will choose a "preponderance" standard. Nevertheless, nothing prevents a legislative body from setting a higher standard for the state to prove that defendants are competent. The mental health expert who is required by statute or encouraged by the trial court to provide an "ultimate opinion" regarding the legal issue of competency should be aware of the standard set by the jurisdiction.

Godinez provides an example of the need to look to the courts for direction about what sort of evidence will be useful. Mental health professionals might expect different standards for different types of competency, but the court applies only one standard - the *Dusky* standard - during the entire process. The clinician who assesses and describes all relevant abilities will likely encounter no difficulty with the court's interpretation of the standard. The evidence is presented, and the court uses this information to reach a decision, regardless of the decision formula it applies. Simply offering an ultimate issue opinion may not be helpful, even if one is required.

Alford provides some insight regarding how the Supreme Court defines rational choice. The focus of the majority was not on the fairness of the choices, but on whether the alternatives were rationally evaluated. The clinician should focus on a defendant's ability to rationally consider choices, regardless of their gravity. The dissent in *Alford* insisted that the nature of the choice amounted to coercion to such an extent that the defendant's choice to plead guilty could not be construed as a voluntary one.

Defendants do not have a right to willfully confuse matters by creating doubts regarding their competency to proceed. In *U.S. v. Greer*, the Court of Appeals for the Fifth Circuit concluded it was appropriate to enhance the sentence of a defendant who feigned mental disorder in order to deceive examiners and the court into believing he was incompetent. To best serve the court, clinicians must offer dispassionate and objective opinions about a defendant's presentation, even though making potentially damaging statements about malingering runs counter to the traditional therapeutic role. Assessing malingering requires a careful examination of the accuracy of the defendant's claims of impairment. Effective examiners avoid acting merely as a conduit for the defendant's "story," and they use whatever tools and techniques are available to discern whether claims of symptoms or deficits are genuine. In *Greer*, the court obtained evidence about malingering from a variety of sources, including mental health professionals, medical professional, correctional staff, and its own observations. Clinicians should verify their impressions that defendants are impaired by consulting those who have observed them in a variety of settings.

Section 4

Incompetent Defendants

Introduction to Section 4

The cases in this section concern issues that arise for incompetent defendants. In *Riggins v. Nevada* (1992), the Supreme Court ruled that it was clear error to try a defendant who had been denied the opportunity to discontinue antipsychotic medication in order to demonstrate his "true mental state" to the jury. The Supreme Court, however, did not address the constitutionality of involuntarily medicating individuals to make them competent to stand trial. Although the Supreme Court had been silent on this issue, the Court of Appeals for the District of Columbia Circuit concluded in *Van Khiem v. United States* (1992) that Van Khiem, charged with murder, could be involuntarily medicated to make him competent. The court held that the government's interest in prosecuting a murder case trumped Van Khiem's right to resist bodily intrusion. This same court echoed that decision in *United States v. Weston* (2001). Additionally, it found that a defendant does not necessarily have a right to reproduce the mental state under which a crime may have been committed. In *United States v. Brandon* (1998), the Court of Appeals for the Sixth Circuit ruled that the degree of bodily intrusion required for involuntary medication necessitated judicial approval, holding that local administrative review was insufficient to safeguard the rights of the defendant, because hospital staff lack judicial training.

The Supreme Court's decision in *Sell v. United States* (2003) delineated issues which must be addressed when medication is indicated solely for competency restoration. The Supreme Court emphasized that the potential contributions and liabilities of medication related to trial competencies should be thoroughly detailed and addressed in any such requests.

In *Jackson v. Indiana* (1972), the Supreme Court held that "due process requires that the nature and duration of commitment have some reasonable relation to the purpose for which the individual is committed." As such, continued commitment must be warranted by progress toward a treatment goal. Because there was no prospect for Jackson to become competent, his commitment for the purpose of competency restoration treatment was unjust. In *United States v. Duhon*, a trial court judge rejected progress reports from a psychoeducational "competency restoration group" as valid or reliable evidence of competency to proceed.

Riggins v. Nevada

504 U.S. 127 (1992)

Facts

David Riggins was arrested for murder in November 1987. Shortly after being taken into custody, he reported symptoms of auditory hallucinations and sleep disturbance. He told a psychiatrist that he had been effectively treated with the antipsychotic medication Mellaril in the past. A prescription for Mellaril was initiated and gradually increased to 800 mg daily. In early 1988, Riggins underwent three competency evaluations. Two of three psychiatrists believed he was competent to proceed, and the district court ruled he was competent. In June 1988, the defense argued that the forced administration of Mellaril and Dilantin infringed on Riggins' freedom by altering his thought processes. Defense counsel argued that the medications would "hide" his "true mental state" at trial, thereby denying him due process of law. Following an evidentiary hearing, the court denied his motion to discontinue the medication. At trial, Riggins pled not guilty by reason of insanity and testified in his own defense. He was convicted and sentenced to death.

Procedural History

On appeal to the Nevada Supreme Court, Riggins argued that forced medication prejudicially affected his attitude, appearance, and demeanor at trial. Furthermore, he contended that the state failed to demonstrate a need for the medication and failed to explore alternatives to psychiatric medication. The Nevada Supreme Court affirmed the conviction, explaining that expert testimony at trial was sufficient to inform the jury of the effect of the psychiatric medications on Riggins' presentation.

Issue

Does forced administration of antipsychotic medication to a defendant during trial violate rights guaranteed by the Sixth and Fourteenth Amendments?[1]

---

[1] Sixth and Fourteenth Amendments. See Appendix B (pp. 261-262).

Holding

The forced administration of antipsychotic medication during trial violates a defendant's Sixth and Fourteenth Amendment rights absent a finding of the need for medication, a finding as to its medical appropriateness, consideration of reasonable alternatives, and consideration of the possible bias against the defendant.

Analysis

The trial court failed to recognize that Riggins had a liberty interest, that is, an interest in being free from unwanted psychiatric medications. In *Washington v. Harper*, the Supreme Court found it impermissible to forcibly medicate a convicted prisoner in the absence of overriding justification and a determination that the medication was necessary. Accordingly, the Fourteenth Amendment[2] affords "at least that much protection" to criminal defendants. Thus, once Riggins moved to terminate administration of antipsychotic medication, the state became obligated to establish the need for the medication and its medical appropriateness. However, the district court allowed Riggins' forced medication to continue without making any determination of the need for the medication or any finding about reasonable alternatives.

Additionally, the U.S. Supreme Court expressed concern that Riggins' defense may have been hindered by the imposition of medication, as the treatment may have adversely affected his outward appearance, his ability to follow the proceedings, the content of his testimony, and the substance of his communication with counsel. The substantial probability of trial prejudice can be justified in some circumstances, such as when it is necessary to guarantee the accomplishment of some essential state function, such as criminal prosecution. In such cases, however, a specific finding is necessary to justify the potential prejudicial effect of psychiatric medication during trial. The record in Riggins contained no finding to support a conclusion that administration of medication was necessary to accomplish an essential state function. Had there been a finding that treatment with an antipsychotic medication was medically appropriate and, considering less intrusive alternatives, was essential for the sake of Riggins' or others' safety, due process would have been satisfied. The ruling of the Nevada Supreme Court was reversed and remanded.

---

[2] Fourteenth Amendment. See Appendix B (p. 262).

Edited Excerpts[3]

David Riggins, Petitioner v. Nevada

Supreme Court of the United States

Certiorari to the Supreme Court of Nevada

504 U.S. 127

May 18, 1992

Justice O'Connor delivered the opinion of the Court, in which Rehnquist, C.J., and White, Blackmun, Stevens, and Souter, JJ., joined. Kennedy, J., filed an opinion concurring in the judgment. Thomas, J. filed a dissenting opinion, in which Scalia, J., joined in part.

During the early hours of November 20, 1987, Paul Wade was found dead in his Las Vegas apartment. An autopsy revealed that Wade died from multiple stab wounds, including wounds to the head, chest, and back. David Riggins was arrested for the killing 45 hours later. A few days after being taken into custody, Riggins told Dr. R. Edward Quass, a private psychiatrist who treated patients at the Clark County Jail, about hearing voices in his head and having trouble sleeping. Riggins informed Dr. Quass that he had been successfully treated with Mellaril in the past. Mellaril is the trade name for thioridazine, an antipsychotic drug. After this consultation, Dr. Quass prescribed Mellaril at a level of 100 milligrams per day. Because Riggins continued to complain of voices and sleep problems in the following months, Dr. Quass gradually increased the Mellaril prescription to 800 milligrams per day. Riggins also received a prescription for Dilantin, an antiepileptic drug.

> **Riggins also asserted that, because he would offer an insanity defense at trial, he had a right to show jurors his "true mental state."**

In January 1988, Riggins successfully moved for a determination of his competence to stand trial. Three court-appointed psychiatrists performed examinations during February and March, while Riggins was taking 450 milligrams of Mellaril daily. Dr.

---

[3] Readers are advised to quote only from the original published cases. See pages vii-viii.

William O'Gorman, a psychiatrist who had treated Riggins for anxiety in 1982, and Dr. Franklin Master concluded that Riggins was competent to stand trial. The third psychiatrist, Dr. Jack Jurasky, found that Riggins was incompetent. The Clark County District Court determined that Riggins was legally sane and competent to stand trial, so preparations for trial went forward.

In early June, the defense moved the District Court for an order suspending administration of Mellaril and Dilantin until the end of Riggins' trial. Relying on both the Fourteenth Amendment and the Nevada Constitution, Riggins argued that continued administration of these drugs infringed upon his freedom and that the drugs' effect on his demeanor and mental state during trial would deny him due process. Riggins also asserted that, because he would offer an insanity defense at trial, he had a right to show jurors his "true mental state." In response, the State noted that Nevada law prohibits the trial of incompetent persons and argued that the court therefore had authority to compel Riggins to take medication necessary to ensure his competence.

On July 14, 1988, the District Court held an evidentiary hearing on Riggins' motion. At the hearing, Dr. Master "guessed" that taking Riggins off medication would not noticeably alter his behavior or render him incompetent to stand trial. Dr. Quass testified that, in his opinion, Riggins would be competent to stand trial even without the administration of Mellaril, but that the effects of Mellaril would not be noticeable to jurors if medication continued. Finally, Dr. O'Gorman told the court that Mellaril made the defendant calmer and more relaxed but that an excessive dose would cause drowsiness. Dr. O'Gorman was unable to predict how Riggins might behave if taken off antipsychotic medication, yet he questioned the need to give Riggins the high dose he was receiving. The court also had before it a written report in which Dr. Jurasky held to his earlier view that Riggins was incompetent to stand

> **The court did not acknowledge the defendant's liberty interest in freedom from unwanted antipsychotic drugs.**

trial and predicted that if taken off Mellaril the defendant "would most likely regress to a manifest psychosis and become extremely difficult to manage."

The District Court denied Riggins' motion to terminate medication with a one-page order that gave no indication of the court's rationale. Riggins continued to receive 800 milligrams of Mellaril each day through the completion of his trial the following November. At trial, Riggins presented an insanity defense and testified on his own behalf. He indicated that on the night of

Wade's death he used cocaine before going to Wade's apartment. Riggins admitted fighting with Wade, but claimed that Wade was trying to kill him and that voices in his head said that killing Wade would be justifiable homicide. A jury found Riggins guilty of murder with use of a deadly weapon and robbery with use of a deadly weapon. After a penalty hearing, the same jury set the murder sentence at death.

Riggins presented several claims to the Nevada Supreme Court, among them that forced administration of Mellaril denied him the ability to assist in his own defense and prejudicially affected his attitude, appearance, and demeanor at trial. We granted *certiorari* to decide whether forced administration of antipsychotic medication during trial violated rights guaranteed by the Sixth and Fourteenth Amendments.

The parties have indicated that once the District Court denied Riggins' motion to terminate use of Mellaril, subsequent administration of the drug was involuntary. This understanding accords with the determination of the Nevada Supreme Court. We also presume that administration of Mellaril was medically appropriate. Finally, the record is dispositive with respect to Riggins' Eighth Amendment claim that administration of Mellaril denied him an opportunity to show jurors his true mental condition at the sentencing hearing.

In *Harper*, a prison inmate alleged that the State of Washington and various individuals violated his right to due process by giving him Mellaril and other antipsychotic drugs against his will. Although the inmate did not prevail, we agreed that his interest in avoiding involuntary administration of antipsychotic drugs was protected under the Fourteenth Amendment's Due Process Clause. "The forcible injection of medication into a nonconsenting person's body," we said, "represents a substantial interference with that person's liberty." Under *Harper*, forcing antipsychotic drugs on a convicted prisoner is impermissible absent a finding of overriding justifica-

> **What the testimony of doctors who examined Riggins establishes, and what we will not ignore, is a strong possibility that Riggins' defense was impaired due to the administration of Mellaril.**

tion and a determination of medical appropriateness. The Fourteenth Amendment affords at least as much protection to persons the State detains for trial. Thus, once Riggins moved to terminate administration of antipsychotic medication, the State became obligated to establish the need for Mellaril and the medical appropriateness of the drug.

Although we have not had occasion to develop substantive standards for judging forced administration of such drugs in the trial or pretrial settings, Nevada certainly would have satisfied due process if the prosecution had demonstrated, and the District Court had found, that treatment with antipsychotic medication was medically appropriate and, considering less intrusive alternatives, essential for the sake of Riggins' own safety or the safety of others. Similarly, the State might have been able to justify medically appropriate, involuntary treatment with the drug by establishing that it could not obtain an adjudication of Riggins' guilt or innocence by using less intrusive means. The question whether a competent criminal defendant may refuse antipsychotic medication if cessation of medication would render him incompetent at trial is not before us.

The court's laconic order denying Riggins' motion did not adopt the State's view, which was that continued administration of Mellaril was required to ensure that the defendant could be tried; in fact, the hearing testimony casts considerable doubt on that argument. Nor did the order indicate a finding that safety considerations or other compelling concerns outweighed Riggins' interest in freedom from unwanted antipsychotic drugs. Were we to divine the District Court's logic from the hearing transcript, we would have to conclude that the court simply weighed the risk that the defense would be prejudiced by changes in Riggins' outward appearance against the chance that Riggins would become incompetent if taken off Mellaril, and struck the balance in favor of involuntary medication. The court did not acknowledge the defendant's liberty interest in freedom from unwanted antipsychotic drugs. This error may well have impaired the constitutionally protected trial rights Riggins invokes. Like the consequences of compelling a defendant to wear prison clothing or of binding and gagging an accused during trial, the precise consequences of forcing antipsychotic medication upon Riggins cannot be shown from a trial transcript. What the testimony of doctors who examined Riggins establishes, and what we will not ignore, is a strong possibility that Riggins' defense was impaired due to the administration of Mellaril.

We also are persuaded that allowing Riggins to present expert testimony about the effect of Mellaril on his demeanor did nothing to cure the possibility that the substance of his own testimony, his interaction with counsel, or his comprehension at trial were compromised by forced administration of Mellaril. Because the record contains no finding that might support a conclusion that administration of antipsychotic medication was necessary to accomplish an essential state policy, however, we have no basis for saying that the substantial probability of trial prejudice in this case was justified.

Justice Kennedy, Concurring in the Judgment

I file this separate opinion, however, to express my view that absent an extraordinary showing by the State, the Due Process Clause prohibits prosecuting officials from administering involuntary doses of antipsychotic medicines for purposes of rendering the accused competent for trial, and to express doubt that the showing can be made in most cases, given our present understanding of the properties of these drugs. It is a fundamental

> *It is a fundamental assumption of the adversary system that the trier of fact observes the accused throughout the trial. (Kennedy, concurring)*

assumption of the adversary system that the trier of fact observes the accused throughout the trial, while the accused is either on the stand or sitting at the defense table. This assumption derives from the right to be present at trial, which in turn derives from the right to testify and rights under the Confrontation Clause.[4] At all stages of the proceedings, the defendant's behavior, manner, facial expressions, and emotional responses, or their absence, combine to make an overall impression on the trier of fact, an impression that can have a powerful influence on the outcome of the trial. If the defendant takes the stand, as Riggins did, his demeanor can have a great bearing on his credibility and persuasiveness, and on the degree to which he evokes sympathy. The defendant's demeanor may also be relevant to his confrontation rights.

The side effects of antipsychotic drugs may alter demeanor in a way that will prejudice all facets of the defense. Serious due process concerns are implicated when the State manipulates the evidence in this way. Concerns about medication extend also to the issue of cooperation with counsel. We have held that a defendant's right to the effective assistance of counsel is impaired when he cannot cooperate in an active manner with his lawyer. The defendant must be able to provide needed information to his lawyer and to participate in the making of decisions on his own behalf.

---

[4] Sixth Amendment, Confrontation Clause. See Appendix B (pp. 261-262).

The side effects of antipsychotic drugs can hamper the attorney-client relation, preventing effective communication and rendering the defendant less able or willing to take part in his defense. The State interferes with this relation when it administers a drug to dull cognition.

If the State cannot render the defendant competent without involuntary medication, then it must resort to civil commitment, if appropriate, unless the defendant becomes competent through other means. If the defendant cannot be tried without his behavior and demeanor being affected in this substantial way by involuntary treatment, in my view the Constitution requires that society bear this cost in order to preserve the integrity of the trial process.

Justice Thomas, With Whom Justice Scalia Joins [in Part], Dissenting

The Court's opinion, in my view, conflates two distinct questions: whether Riggins had a full and fair criminal trial and whether Nevada improperly forced Riggins to take medication. In this criminal case, Riggins is asking, and may ask, only for the reversal of his conviction and sentence. He is not seeking, and may not seek, an injunction to terminate his medical treatment or damages for an infringement of his personal rights. I agree with the positions of the majority and concurring opinions in the Nevada Supreme Court: Even if the State truly forced Riggins to take medication, and even if this medication deprived Riggins of a protected liberty interest in a manner actionable in a different legal proceeding, Riggins nonetheless had the fundamentally fair criminal trial required by the Constitution. I therefore would affirm his conviction.

> *If the defendant cannot be tried without his behavior and demeanor being affected by involuntary treatment, the Constitution requires that society bear this cost in order to preserve the integrity of the trial process. (Kennedy, concurring)*

Riggins contended in the Nevada Supreme Court that he did not have a "full and fair trial" for two reasons, the first relating to exclusion of evidence of his mental condition and the second concerning his ability to assist in his defense.

The Court fails to explain why the medication's effects rendered Riggins' trial fundamentally unfair. The trial court offered Riggins the opportunity to prove his mental condition as it existed at the time of the crime through testimony instead of his appearance in court in an unmedicated condition. Riggins took advantage of this offer by explaining to the jury the history of his mental health, his usage of Mellaril, and the possible effects of Mellaril on his demeanor. Riggins also called Dr. Jack A. Jurasky, a psychiatrist, who testified about Riggins' condition after his arrest and his likely mental state at the time of the crime. Dr. Jurasky also explained Riggins' use of Mellaril and how it might be affecting him. The Nevada Supreme Court concluded that this "testimony was sufficient to inform the jury of the effect of the Mellaril on Riggins' demeanor and testimony."

Riggins also argued in the Nevada Supreme Court, although not in his briefs to this Court, that he did not have a "full and fair trial" because Mellaril had side effects that interfered with his ability to participate in his defense. Riggins has no claim of legal incompetence in this case. The trial court specifically found him competent while he was taking Mellaril under a statute requiring him to have "sufficient mentality to be able to understand the nature of the criminal charges against him, and to aid and assist his counsel in the defense interposed upon the trial."

Riggins also argues for reversal on the basis of our holding in *Washington v. Harper* that the Due Process Clause protects a substantive "liberty interest" in avoiding unwanted medication. Riggins asserts that Nevada unconstitutionally deprived him of this liberty interest by forcing him to take Mellaril. Riggins may not complain about a deprivation of the liberty interest that we recognized in *Harper* because the record does not support his version of the facts. Shortly after his arrest, as the Court notes, Riggins told a psychiatrist at his jail that he was hearing voices and could not sleep. The psychiatrist prescribed Mellaril. When the prescription did not eliminate the problem, Riggins sought further treatment and the psychiatrist increased the dosage. Riggins thus began taking the drug voluntarily. The Court concludes that the medication became involuntary when the trial

> *I do not mean to suggest that States may drug detainees at their whim. (Thomas, dissenting)*

court denied Riggins' motion for permission not to take the drug during the trial. I disagree. Although the court denied Riggins' motion, it did not order him to take any medication.

Finally, we did not grant *certiorari*[5] to determine whether the Nevada courts had made the findings required by *Harper* to sup-

---

[5] *certiorari.* A means of gaining appellate review.

port forced administration of a drug. We took this case to decide
"whether forced medication during trial violates a defendant's
constitutional right to a full and fair trial." The Court declines to
answer this question one way or the other, stating only that a violation of *Harper* "may well have impaired the constitutionally
protected trial rights Riggins invokes." As we have stated, "we
ordinarily do not consider questions outside those presented in
the petition for *certiorari*." I believe that we should refuse to consider Riggins' *Harper* argument.

I do not mean in any way to undervalue the importance of a
person's liberty interest in avoiding forced medication or to suggest that States may drug detainees at their whim. Under
Harper, detainees have an interest in avoiding unwanted medication that the States must respect. In appropriate instances, detainees may seek damages or injunctions against further medication in civil actions. Yet, when this Court reviews a state-court
criminal conviction of a defendant who has taken medication, it
cannot undo any violation that already has occurred or punish
those responsible. It may determine only whether the defendant
received a proper trial, free of the kinds of reversible errors that
we have recognized. Because Riggins had a full and fair trial in
this case, I would affirm the Nevada Supreme Court.

Van Khiem v. United States

612 A.2d 160 (1992)

Facts

60-year-old Tran Van Khiem was charged with murdering his parents in 1986. His behavior in court was so bizarre that a competency evaluation was ordered. He was found not competent and hospitalized at St. Elizabeth's Hospital in Washington, DC. He refused to take psychiatric medications voluntarily, and for several years, the hospital chose not to medicate him against his will, as there was some disagreement regarding whether medications would benefit him. In 1989, the prosecution sought to have him medicated by force. The hospital assigned a new psychiatrist who believed such treatment could reduce his psychotic symptoms and possibly restore him to competency. Van Khiem resisted, first through St. Elizabeth's internal review procedure, then through two judicial hearings. When a judge ordered forced medication, he appealed.

Issue

Can a defendant be medicated against his or her will in an effort to restore competency to stand trial?

Holding

The Court of Appeals affirmed the trial court's decision to forcibly medicate Van Khiem. This defendant argued that forced administration of psychiatric medication violated his right to bodily integrity. The court ruled that such intrusion is permissible if there is overriding justification and if it is medically appropriate. Once such a showing is made, the patient enjoys due process protection only if the determination is found to be arbitrary or unreasonable. Van Khiem argued the treatment was arbitrary because it was not based solely on his medical interests. However, *Washington v. Harper* demonstrated that the patient's interests are not necessarily primary. It made no sense to withhold the very treatment for which Van Khiem was committed.

Analysis

This decision underscored that the right to reject medical treatment is not absolute. Van Khiem argued that the prosecution must demonstrate that its interest in forcing medication is compelling and that no reasonable alternative exists. The court ruled that although alternatives should be considered, the government is not compelled to explore and reject every conceivable alternative.

The government has a compelling interest in trying those accused of violating the law. The government's interest in forcibly medicating an individual to restore him or her to competency is therefore fundamental and of very high order. At this time (just on the heels of the Supreme Court Case of *Riggins v. Nevada*), most courts upheld the ability to medicate patients by force when necessary. Patients were protected only from arbitrary and capricious state action.

Edited Excerpts[1]

Tran Van Khiem, Appellant, v. United States, et al., Appellees

District of Columbia Court of Appeals

612 A.2d 160

August 18, 1992

Before Schwelb and Wagner, Associate Judges, and Gallagher, Senior Judge

Schwelb, Associate Judge

Tran Van Khiem (Khiem) was charged in 1986 with the premeditated murder of his parents. He was found incompetent to stand trial and is presently detained at Saint Elizabeth's Hospital (the hospital). He now appeals from an order of the trial court directing that he be treated, over his objection, with psychotropic drugs. The primary purpose of the proposed treatment would be to render Khiem competent to stand trial. Khiem contends that the administration of these drugs to him without his consent

---

[1] Readers are advised to quote only from the original published cases. See pages vii-viii.

would abrogate his common-law right to bodily integrity. He also claims that the standards and procedures utilized by the hospital and by the trial judge in ordering treatment run afoul of the Due Process Clause of the Fifth Amendment.[2] We hold that the trial court made a reasonable accommodation between Khiem's liberty interest and the government's interest in bringing him to trial, and that the procedures utilized below satisfied applicable constitutional standards. Accordingly, we affirm.

On the morning of July 24, 1986, the bodies of Mr. Tran Van Chuong and Mrs. Nam Tran Chuong, an elderly couple who were members of a prominent Vietnamese family, were found in their home in northwest Washington, DC. Investigation disclosed that both Chuongs had died from asphyxiation and that each had apparently been severely beaten. On July 25, 1986, their son, appellant Tran Van Khiem, then sixty years of age, was arrested and charged with the murders. Khiem was detained at the District of Columbia Jail. An indictment was returned on April 22, 1987, charging Khiem with two counts of murder in the first degree.

On June 25, 1987, following preliminary proceedings in which Khiem indicated that he did not propose to offer an insanity defense, Chief Judge Fred Ugast ordered that Khiem be transferred to the hospital for an examination of his mental condition. He directed the hospital to determine whether Khiem was competent to stand trial, whether an insanity defense might be available to him, and, if so, whether Khiem was competent to waive it. Following several examinations and communications with the court, the hospital reported that Khiem was competent to stand trial and that he did not qualify for an insanity defense. The trial was rescheduled for March 8, 1988 and began on that date. As the trial proceeded, Khiem conducted himself in a bizarre manner.[3] At the request of defense counsel, Judge Ugast halted the proceedings and ordered a competency screening. On March 18, 1988, after hearing testimony from the examining psychiatrist, the judge found Khiem incompetent to stand trial. The judge declared a mistrial and recommitted him to the hospital for evaluation and treatment. The purpose of the commitment was to enable Khiem to regain his trial competency.

On June 13, 1988, the hospital reported that Khiem was incompetent to stand trial and that he was unlikely to regain his competency in the foreseeable future. This diagnosis was repeated on several occasions over the following two years at proceedings

---

[2] Due Process Clause of the Fifth Amendment. See Appendix B (p. 261).

[3] Khiem is reported to suffer from paranoid delusions about world-wide conspiracies related to him and his parents.

convened by the trial court. A psychiatrist who had examined Khiem on behalf of the prosecution suggested at a 1989 hearing that antipsychotic medication could have some potential for improving Khiem's condition and restoring his competency for trial. Judge Robert Shuker, to whom the case had been reassigned, directed the hospital to explore this possibility. The hospital advised the court, however, by letter dated September 18, 1989, that it had decided that psychotropic medication should not be administered to Khiem on an involuntary basis. It was the view of Dr. John Kelley, the Medical Director of the John Howard Pavilion, that Khiem was unlikely to respond positively to such medication and that his prognosis, with or without medication, was poor. On October 4, 1989, the prosecution filed a motion to require [Khiem's] involuntary medication. The defense responded with a motion to terminate Khiem's commitment. On September 25, 1990, Judge Robert M. Scott, to whom the case had been reassigned, directed the hospital to provide an updated report.

In response to the judge's order, the hospital reported that Khiem remained incompetent. Following an evaluation by his new doctor, Kenneth Rogers, MD, however, the hospital now recommended that Khiem be treated with psychotropic drugs. The hospital indicated that psychotropic medication could reduce the symptoms of Khiem's illness (including his psychotic thinking) and render him competent for trial. Khiem invoked the hospital's internal administrative review procedures in an attempt to have this recommendation set aside. His administrative appeal was unsuccessful and, on March 19, 1991, Dr. Rogers' decision was affirmed by the hospital administration. Khiem, through counsel, asked the trial court not to follow the hospital's recommendation. The trial judge convened two hearings to determine how Khiem's case should proceed.

> *As Khiem interprets it, a criminal defendant may determine unilaterally whether he may be brought to trial.*

On April 11, 1991, after considering the briefs and arguments of counsel, he concluded that the question for his consideration was whether the hospital's recommendation was arbitrary or capricious. Thereafter, at an evidentiary hearing which began on July 29, 1991, the judge received the testimony of one medical witness called on behalf of Khiem and of three medical witnesses - Dr. Rogers, Dr. Kelley, and Dr. John Livingood - called by the prosecution. The government's witnesses testified that the proposed involuntary treatment was medically indicated and that appropriate safeguards would be taken to avert any possible side effects. The psychiatrist called by Khiem disagreed with the hospital's recommendation, but acknowledged that a minority of psychiatrists, especially those who practiced forensic medicine, might agree with the hospital's decision.

The judge ruled that the hospital's recommendation "has been shown to be wholly reasonable and to have been based upon clinical determinations which are well founded medically." He specifically found, contrary to Khiem's claims, that the hospital's treatment decision had not been influenced by a desire to accommodate the perceived wishes of the court or the prosecution. The judge rejected, on the strength of *Washington v. Harper* and *United States v. Charters*, Khiem's contention that the court was without authority to order treatment unless Khiem consented to it, either personally or through the substituted judgment process. The judge authorized the hospital to administer psychotropic medication to Khiem for a sixty-day period, but ordered that the patient be monitored for unfavorable side effects and that the treatment be discontinued if this was necessary to assure Khiem's well-being. The hospital was directed to make a progress report to the court within seventy-five days of the commencement of medication. This appeal followed.

Relying primarily on this court's reference in *In re A.C.* to "the tenet common to all medical treatment cases: that any person has the right to make an informed choice, if competent to do so, to accept or forego medical treatment," Khiem contends that the trial judge's order unlawfully overrode his common-law right to bodily integrity.[4] He claims that before authorizing psychotropic medication, the trial judge was required to make a determination whether Khiem was competent to decide whether such medication should be administered to him. Khiem further maintains that if the judge found him not to be competent to make that decision, then the judge was obliged to apply the principle of substituted judgment to ascertain what Khiem's wishes would have been if he

> *It would surely be incongruous to hold that the court, after committing an accused for treatment to render him competent, is obliged to withhold treatment at the accused's sole option.*

---

[4] In its *amicus* brief urging reversal, the American Civil Liberties Union of the National Capital Area (ACLU) goes further and contends that the trial court's order that psychotropic drugs be administered to Khiem contravened the Due Process Clause of the Fifth Amendment. We are not disposed to broaden the issues beyond those raised in Khiem's behalf by his able counsel from the Public Defender Service.

had been competent to decide. Extracting *A.C.* from its context, Khiem evidently maintains that in light of our decision in that case, trial judges are now without authority, as a matter of local common law, to order any medical treatment over a patient's objection, whether that objection is interposed directly by the patient or indirectly through the substituted judgment process. This rule, according to Khiem, is absolute; the court in *A.C.*, he insists, "recognized no limits on who is protected by this common law principle." Our decision in *A.C.*, as Khiem interprets it, would effectively enable a criminal defendant in his position to determine unilaterally whether he may be brought to trial. We discern nothing in *A.C.* which would support such a one-sided doctrine.

As we indicated in *A.C.*, the common-law liberty interest in one's own bodily integrity is an important one. The Supreme Court, speaking through Chief Justice Rehnquist, recently reiterated its view, initially articulated more than a century ago, that "no right is held more sacred, or is more carefully guarded, by the common law, than the right of every individual to the possession and control of his own person, free from all restraint or interference of others, unless by clear and unquestionable authority of law" (*Cruzan v. Missouri Dep't of Health*). That right embraces a "significant liberty interest in avoiding the unwanted administration of antipsychotic drugs" for "the forcible injection of medication into a nonconsenting person's body represents a substantial interference with that person's liberty" (*Harper*). We also agree with Khiem that his rights under the common law were not extinguished by his commitment to the lawful custody of the hospital. In *Harper*, the Court recognized that a mentally ill individual who has been sentenced to imprisonment retains a right, both under state law and under the Due Process Clause of the Fourteenth Amendment,[5] to be free from the arbitrary administration of antipsychotic medication. But our recognition of this important aspect of individual autonomy in a free society does not lead us to accord it the absolute and preemptive character which Khiem claims for it. The government cannot intrude upon Khiem's bodily integrity without a showing of overriding justification and medical appropriateness (*Riggins*). Once such a showing has been made, however, Khiem enjoys common-law or due process protection only from an unreasonable or arbitrary determination that involuntary medication is appropriate. Khiem's common-law interest, like his due process protections, must be weighed against

---

[5] Due Process Clause of the Fourteenth Amendment. See Appendix B (p. 262).

any legitimate interests asserted by the state, and a reasoned accommodation must be made between the competing interests.[6]

Moreover, Khiem having been lawfully committed to the hospital, the extent of his rights must be assessed in the context of his confinement. The statute under which Khiem was committed, provides that the court may commit an apparently incompetent criminal defendant to a mental hospital for "care and treatment" in order to enable him to regain his competency. It would surely be incongruous to hold that the court, after committing an accused for treatment to render him competent so that he can stand trial for the offenses with which he has been charged, is obliged to withhold treatment at the accused's sole option.

Finally, Khiem contends that the prosecution is required to prove that its interest in medicating him over his objection is so compelling that no reasonable alternative exists. The availability of reasonable alternatives to the proposed treatment, if shown, would be a relevant factor in the overall inquiry, but this does not necessarily mean that the government

> *Constitutional power to bring an accused to trial is fundamental to a scheme of "ordered liberty" and prerequisite to social justice and peace.*

must "set up and then shoot down every conceivable alternative method of accommodating the claimant's constitutional [or common law] complaint" (*Harper*). In any event, as we show below, the law enforcement interest asserted by the government in the present case, which involves two alleged murders, is an especially compelling one.

Having assessed Khiem's liberty interest, we turn now to the competing interest asserted by the United States. As Justice Brennan wrote in his concurring opinion in *Illinois v. Allen*, "the safeguards that the Constitution accords to criminal defendants presuppose that government has a sovereign prerogative to put on trial those accused in good faith of violating valid laws. Constitutional power to bring an accused to trial is fundamental to a scheme of 'ordered liberty' and prerequisite to social justice and peace."[7] Since it has been impossible for several years to bring

---

[6] In *Harper*, the Court explicitly rejected a constitutional contention by a mentally ill prisoner identical to Khiem's common-law claim here: Respondent contends that the State, under the mandate of the Due Process Clause, may not override his choice to refuse antipsychotic drugs unless he has been found to be incompetent, and then only if the factfinder makes a substituted judgment that he, if competent, would consent to drug treatment. We disagree.

[7] Justice Brennan added that if a resolution of criminal charges "cannot be reached by judicial trial in a court of law, it will be reached elsewhere and by

Khiem to trial to determine his guilt or innocence without first administering psychotropic medication, the government's interest is a "fundamental" one and of a very high order indeed. In *Winston v. Lee*, the Court treated as important (though not as controlling) the government's interest in obtaining a bullet from a criminal suspect's chest. That bullet would, however, have represented but one part of the evidence against the defendant. In the present case, it appears to be beyond dispute that if Khiem is not treated with psychotropic medication, the prosecution will not be able to bring him to trial at all. The societal interest at issue is therefore considerably greater than that presented by the government in the bullet recovery cases.

The ACLU argues in its *amicus* brief[8] that the government's interest is "largely symbolic," because even if Khiem is convicted,

> **The government's law enforcement interest outweighs Khiem's interest in bodily integrity.**

"he will in all likelihood return in short order to some form of institutional psychiatric care." We cannot agree with the ACLU's characterization. We note that Khiem has asked the court to terminate his commitment and that he emphatically denies that he is a danger to himself or to anyone else. An individual may not be civilly committed unless it is demonstrated that he is likely to injure himself or others. Accordingly, if all of the declarations on Khiem's behalf were taken at face value, and if his legal contentions were to prevail, he might soon be a free man without his guilt or innocence of two murders having first been established, and this could continue indefinitely unless he regained his competency to stand trial. Unless we view the trial of homicide cases, the deterrence and punishment of crime, and the incapacitation of criminals as insignificant, the government's law enforcement interest in determining whether Khiem murdered his parents is far more than merely symbolic.

Although the issue does not appear to have been squarely decided in this jurisdiction, most of the courts which have been asked to do so have upheld the involuntary administration of psychotropic drugs to restore or maintain a defendant's competency for trial. In holding that the hospital may treat Khiem with such medication without his consent, the trial judge relied not only on

---

other means, and there will be grave danger that liberty, equality, and the order essential to both will be lost."

[8] *amicus* brief. A legal paper submitted to the court by a person or party not involved in the case, usually arguing for a certain outcome, or intended to call the court's attention to some matter.

Harper but also on *Charters*. In *Charters*, the United States Court of Appeals for the Fourth Circuit, sitting *en banc*,[9] affirmed a trial court order authorizing the involuntary treatment with psychotropic medication of a mentally ill defendant who had been indicted for allegedly threatening the President of the United States. Charters had been found incompetent and committed to a prison mental health facility for psychiatric examination and treatment. The court held that although an individual so committed was not thereby stripped of all of his liberty interests, those interests which he retained were afforded protection only against arbitrary and capricious state action, and were adequately secured by the exercise of the professional judgment of the prison facility's medical personnel. The court recognized that the government's interest in maintaining a pretrial detainee in a competent condition to stand trial was a "legitimate incident of institutionalization" to which Charters' interest must yield.[10]

Accordingly, we reject Khiem's common-law claim.

In the present case, as in *Harper* and *Charters*, an informed medical judgment on the benefits and risks of the proposed treatment is central to the weighing and accommodation of the competing interests, and the reasoning of the courts in *Harper* and *Charters* applies in full measure.[11] Even if we were to conclude, contrary to the quoted passages from *Harper* and *Charters*, that the "societal and legal implications" of the issue before the trial judge warranted less deference to the hospital's recommendation than the judge accorded it, any error would not be prejudicial to Khiem. The trial court obviously recognized the importance of the government's law enforcement interest; indeed, it was Judge Shuker's allusion to that interest that set in motion the events which culminated in the entry by Judge Scott of the order

---

[9] *en banc*. All the judges of an appellate court considering an opinion together.

[10] Although we have focused in this opinion on the law enforcement interest in restoring Khiem's competence, there was also evidence before the trial judge which would support a finding that his order served other legitimate purposes. Dr. Kelley testified that Khiem's condition had deteriorated, that his delusions were expanding, and that he (Dr. Kelley) was concerned that, without psychotropic treatment, Khiem (who had already allegedly killed his parents) might strike out against others. (See *Harper*.) Dr. Livingood was of the opinion that medication was now appropriate "because the man does have a psychotic disorder and the treatment offers a chance to help the psychotic disorder and help him become more healthy."

[11] Indeed, Khiem implicitly acknowledges in his brief that his position cannot be reconciled with *Charters*, but suggests that *Charters* has been effectively overruled by the Supreme Court's later decision in *Harper*. We discern no inconsistency between *Harper* and *Charters*; indeed, the two decisions point us in the same direction.

now on appeal. Moreover, if the decision as to the weight to be accorded to that interest is a legal one, as Khiem suggests, then it is ultimately one that this court must make. Realistically, we have already made it, for we have held in this opinion that on this record, the government's law enforcement interest outweighs Khiem's interest in bodily integrity, especially in light of the safeguards for which the trial court's order provides.[12] Khiem asks us to remand the case but, under these circumstances, a remand would serve no useful purpose. As we recently had occasion to observe *en banc*, "to remand the case simply for the purpose of requiring the judge to make the prescribed finding now would be a symbolic rather than a practical act, which we view as unnecessary and as incompatible with good judicial husbandry."

It is true, as Khiem points out, that the procedure at issue in *Harper* included an adversarial hearing. The Court gave no indication, however, that such a hearing was constitutionally required. Indeed, in *Parham v. J.R.*, the Supreme Court held in a somewhat comparable context that, although such a hearing may be required as a matter of state law, "due process is not violated by the use of informal, traditional medical investigative techniques." In *Charters*, the court, relying on *Parham*, explicitly held that no adversarial hearing is constitutionally required.[13] We reach the same conclusion in this case.

Khiem contends that the hospital's decision was arbitrary because, according to him, no doctor has testified, to a reasonable degree of medical certainty, that the proposed treatment will probably render Mr. Khiem competent to stand trial. He apparently bases this contention on *Jackson v.*

> This is not a case in which a court authorized the hospital to perform complex brain surgery on an individual charged with disorderly conduct.

Indiana. Jackson does not support his claim. The question in *Jackson* was whether a criminal defendant may be committed indefinitely solely on account of his lack of capacity to stand trial. The Court held that a person so detained "cannot be held more than the reasonable period of time necessary to determine whether there is a substantial probability that he will attain that

---

[12] In *Harper*, the Court noted that in the overwhelming majority of cases, judges and other outside decision makers have concurred in the treating physician's decision to treat a patient involuntarily, and that the practical effect of requiring the decision to be made initially by a judge may thus be "chimerical."

[13] The court said: "Making an acceptable professional judgment of the sort here in issue does not require any internal adversarial hearing."

capacity in the foreseeable future." In the absence of a showing of such a substantial probability, the defendant must be released or civil commitment proceedings must be instituted. This eminently sensible holding provides no support for Khiem's claim that physicians may not inaugurate a course of treatment without advance assurance of probable success. Indeed, *Jackson* addressed neither the question of involuntary medication nor the scope of a court's review of medical judgments. In *Harper*, on the other hand, the Supreme Court held that the proper standard for reviewing governmental conduct in this kind of situation is to determine its reasonableness.

Khiem also contends that the hospital's treatment decision must fail the test of rationality and lack of arbitrariness because the decision by the hospital's medical personnel was not made exclusively in the patient's medical interest. In *Harper*, however, the court made it clear that the determination whether to medicate does not turn exclusively on the patient's interests, but also requires consideration of legitimate state interests. The government's law enforcement interest in this case is a significant one, and we hold that it was proper to consider it. This is not a case in which a court authorized the hospital to perform complex brain surgery on an individual charged with disorderly conduct. Rather, the hospital has recommended psychotropic treatment of limited duration, which is to be closely monitored, to permit a determination through the judicial process as to whether Khiem committed two premeditated murders. The judge heard medical testimony which, if credited by him, established that the proposed treatment was consistent with sound medical practice. His decision to follow the hospital's recommendation was neither arbitrary nor irrational.

For the foregoing reasons, the order appealed from is hereby Affirmed.

United States v. Weston

255 F.3d 873 (2001)

Facts

On July 24, 1998, an assailant armed with a .38 caliber revolver forced his way past security checkpoints at the U.S. Capitol. He shot and killed two officers of the U.S. Capitol Police, and
shot and wounded one other. Russell Eugene Weston, seriously
wounded by gunfire, was arrested at the scene and charged with
murder. The government was unable to bring Weston to trial on
these charges because a district court adjudicated him incompetent to stand trial. The district court accepted the conclusion of a
court-appointed forensic psychiatrist that Weston suffered from
paranoid schizophrenia, and that the undisputed severity of his
symptoms rendered him incapable of understanding the proceedings against him and assisting in his defense. Consequently, Weston was committed to the custody of the Federal Correctional Institution in Butner, North Carolina (FCI Butner). While there, he
was "placed in solitary confinement under constant observation"
in an effort to mitigate his dangerousness. It was subsequently
agreed by all parties that antipsychotic medication was likely the
only treatment that might mitigate Weston's schizophrenic symptoms and restore him to competency to stand trial.

Procedural History

While at FCI Butner, Weston received no antipsychotic medication because, at a time when he was considered medically competent to consent to psychiatric medications, he had refused to do
so. Further, the district court prohibited the Bureau of Prisons
(BOP) from forcibly medicating him without a court order. After
two administrative hearings and two district court hearings, the
government obtained an order authorizing administration of antipsychotic medication to Weston over his objections. The district
court found that forcible medication was "medically appropriate"
and "essential for Weston's safety and the safety of others." The
Court of Appeals for the District of Columbia Circuit reversed and
remanded. On remand, the district court again held that the BOP
could forcibly medicate Weston, concluding that antipsychotic
medication was medically appropriate, and essential to control

and treat his dangerousness to others. The district court also found that the government had an essential interest in bringing Weston to trial, given "the serious and violent nature of the charges, that the immediate victims were federal law enforcement officers performing their official duties, and that the killings took place inside the U.S. Capitol amid a crowd of innocent bystanders." Weston again appealed to the Court of Appeals for the District of Columbia Circuit.

Issue

May the government administer unwanted antipsychotic medication to a pretrial detainee in order to render him competent to stand trial?

Holding

The government's interest in administering antipsychotic medication to make Weston competent for trial overrides his liberty interest, and restoring his competence in such a manner does not necessarily violate his right to a fair trial.

Analysis

Under the Due Process Clause of the Fifth Amendment, a pretrial detainee has a significant liberty interest in avoiding the unwanted administration of antipsychotic medication. While this liberty interest is "significant," it is not absolute. In *Washington v. Harper*, the U.S. Supreme Court held that the government may, under certain circumstances, forcibly administer antipsychotic medication to a prisoner or criminal defendant despite his liberty interest, provided such treatment is medically appropriate. A pretrial detainee's liberty interest in avoiding unwanted antipsychotic medication is trumped when the medication is essential to mitigate the detainee's dangerousness. In the present case, the district court measured the medical appropriateness of antipsychotic medication by weighing the capacity of such medication to alleviate Weston's schizophrenic symptoms against its capacity to produce harm (i.e., side effects). The court concluded that the administration of antipsychotic medication to Weston was medically appropriate.

In determining whether a governmental interest overrides a constitutional right, courts must examine not only the nature of the right and the strength of the countervailing interest, but also the fit between the interest and the means chosen to accomplish it. This inquiry entails a predictive judgment about the probable efficacy of the means to satisfy the interest.

In the present case, in order to medicate Weston, the government is required to prove that restoring his competency to stand trial is necessary to accomplish an essential state policy. While it has not been determined under what circumstances trying and punishing offenders is or is not "essential," the court noted that the government's interest in finding, convicting, and punishing criminals "reaches its zenith when the crime is the murder of federal police officers."

Regarding Weston's right to a fair trial, the court noted that a defendant does not have an absolute right to replicate on the witness stand his mental state at the time of the crime.

Edited Excerpts[1]

United States of America, Appellee, v. Russell Eugene Weston, Appellant

Appeal from the United States District Court for the District of Columbia

255 F.3d 873

July 27, 2001

Before Sentelle, Randolph, and Rogers, Circuit Judges

Opinion for the Court Filed by
Circuit Judge Randolph

Under the Fifth Amendment's Due Process Clause there is a "significant liberty interest in avoiding the unwanted administration of antipsychotic drugs" (*Harper*). This appeal requires us to decide whether the government may administer such drugs to a pretrial detainee against his will in order to render him competent to stand trial.

On July 24, 1998, an assailant armed with a .38 caliber revolver forced his way past security checkpoints at the United States Capitol. He shot and killed Jacob Chestnut and John Gibson, both officers of the United States Capitol Police. He shot and seriously wounded Douglas McMillan, also an officer of the

---

[1] Readers are advised to quote only from the original published cases. See pages vii-viii.

United States Capitol Police. Russell Eugene Weston, himself seriously wounded by gunfire, was arrested at the scene. The federal government indicted Weston on two counts of murdering a federal law enforcement officer, one count of attempting to murder a federal law enforcement officer, and three counts of using a firearm in a crime of violence. The government wants to try Weston for these crimes but is presently unable to do so because the district court found him incompetent to stand trial. The district court accepted the conclusion of a court-appointed forensic psychiatrist that Weston suffers from paranoid schizophrenia, and that the severity of his symptoms renders him incapable of understanding the proceedings against him and assisting in his defense, as required to bring a defendant to trial.

The court committed Weston to the custody of the Attorney General "for treatment in a suitable facility for a reasonable period of time." Weston is currently incarcerated "for treatment" at the Federal Correctional Institute in Butner, North Carolina. He is not being treated. Rather, he was placed in solitary confinement under constant observation when he arrived at FCI Butner and remains there today. The Bureau of Prisons apparently placed him in seclusion to "mitigate [his] dangerousness." As an Assistant Director of the Bureau explained, Weston's "mental health seclusion status" is "for very vulnerable inmates, and is typically reserved for those who present a substantial danger to themselves or somebody else." The district court characterized Weston's confinement situation as "simply the warehousing of Weston in a psychotic state. It is not treatment; at best it contains dangerousness." There is treatment available for Weston's illness and its symptoms in the form of antipsychotic medication. The parties agree that such medication is likely the only treatment that can mitigate his schizophrenia and attendant delusions, and thus restore his competence to stand trial. Weston is not currently receiving any such medication because, at a time when he was considered medically competent to make a determination, he refused them. The district court prohibited the Bureau of Prisons from forcibly medicating Weston without a court order.

After two administrative hearings and two district court hearings, the government obtained an order authorizing it to adminis-

> **The court concluded that forcible medication would not interfere with Weston's right to a fair trial, and could in some respects enhance his ability to exercise that right by improving his mental function.**

ter antipsychotic medication against Weston's will. The district court held that forcible medication was "medically appropriate" and "essential for [Weston's] own safety or the safety of others." It also found that "the government has a fundamental interest in bringing the defendant to trial," but determined that the dangerousness holding made it unnecessary to decide whether that interest outweighed Weston's right to refuse antipsychotic medication. The court declined to consider Weston's claim that forced medication would interfere with his right to a fair trial, holding it was not ripe. A panel of this court reversed and remanded the case to the district court, holding that the district court's dangerousness finding was not supported by the record. The panel also reversed the district court's determination that Weston's Sixth Amendment[2] right to a fair trial claim was not ripe, holding that "because antipsychotic medication may affect the defendant's ability to assist in his defense, post-medication review may come too late to prevent impairment of his Sixth Amendment right." The panel also directed the district court to consider Weston's argument that medical ethics preclude forcibly medicating a defendant to make him competent for trial in a case that might carry the death penalty.

On remand, the district court again held that the Bureau of Prisons could forcibly medicate Weston. It concluded that antipsychotic medication was medically appropriate and "essential to control and treat Weston's dangerousness to others." The district court also held that the "government has an essential interest in bringing Weston to trial" given "the serious and violent nature of the charges, that

> **"Weston is simply warehoused in a psychotic state. It is not treatment; at best it contains dangerousness."**

the immediate victims were federal law enforcement officers performing their official duties, and that the killings took place inside the U.S. Capitol amid a crowd of innocent bystanders." The court concluded that forcible medication would not interfere with Weston's right to a fair trial, and could in some respects enhance his ability to exercise that right by improving his mental function.

In this appeal, Weston claims that administering antipsychotic drugs against his will violates his Fifth Amendment[3] due process liberty interest "in avoiding unwanted bodily intrusion" and implicates his right to a fair trial. We affirm the district court's conclusion that the government's interest in administering

---

[2] Sixth Amendment. See Appendix B (pp. 261-262).
[3] Fifth Amendment. See Appendix B (p. 261).

antipsychotic drugs to make Weston competent for trial overrides his liberty interest, and that restoring his competence in such manner does not necessarily violate his right to a fair trial.

The due process liberty interest in avoiding unwanted antipsychotic medication may be "significant," but it is not absolute. In *Harper* and later in *Riggins*, the Supreme Court recognized that the government may, under certain circumstances, forcibly administer antipsychotic medication to a prisoner or criminal defendant despite his liberty interest, provided such medication is "medically appropriate." With respect to Weston, there is no doubt that this latter condition has been met. Whether a proposed course of action is "medically appropriate" obviously depends on the judgment of medical professionals. The district court relied on several experts in concluding that "antipsychotic medication is the medically acceptable and indicated treatment for Weston's illness."

Weston claims that the ethical obligations a doctor owes a patient preclude forcible medication in these circumstances. As he sees it, "The question whether the administration of antipsychotic medication is medically appropriate is different from the question whether treatment is therapeutically appropriate." Thus, "The context in which the forced medication issue arises and the state purpose are relevant considerations for the physician to decide whether it is ethical to force-medicate." If the state's purpose is to make one competent for trial, Weston argues, then a doctor must consider alternatives such as civil

> *No source of legal authority makes medical ethics relevant to the determination whether the government can forcibly medicate Weston.*

commitment. These ethical norms purportedly derive from the Hippocratic Oath and the 1982 United Nations Principles of Medical Ethics Relevant to the Role of Health Personnel, Particularly Physicians, in the Protection of Prisoners and Detainees against Torture, and Other Cruel, Inhuman or Degrading Treatment or Punishment. No source of legal authority - neither Bureau of Prisons regulations, nor the statue governing treatment of incompetent pretrial detainees, nor the Constitution - makes medical ethics relevant to the determination whether the government can forcibly medicate Weston. Even if a particular doctor had ethical objections to administering antipsychotic drugs to a nonconsenting patient, this would not undercut the consensus in the medical profession that antipsychotic medication is the medically appropriate response to Weston's condition.[4]

A pretrial detainee's liberty interest in avoiding unwanted antipsychotic medication gives way when the medication is essential to mitigate the detainee's dangerousness: "Nevada certainly would have satisfied due process if the prosecution had demonstrated, and the District Court had found, that treatment with antipsychotic medication was medically appropriate and, considering less intrusive alternatives, essential for the sake of [the pretrial detainee's] own safety or the safety of others" (*Riggins*). The district court applied this standard to Weston's situation and twice found antipsychotic medication medically appropriate and essential for his safety or the safety of those around him. On appeal of the district court's first decision, a panel of this court found the record insufficient to support application of the *Riggins* standard. Much of the evidence focused on the government's competency-for-trial justification - which the district court did not adopt - and the limited

> **We see little basis to suppose that the jury will take Weston's testimony as an indication that he must have been sane at the time of the crime, or that he is making it up, or that he deserves no sympathy.**

evidence supporting the dangerousness justification "indicates that in his current circumstances Weston poses no significant danger to himself or to others." The panel relied on the testimony of a Public Health Service physician assigned to FCI Butner that "given [Weston's] immediate containment situation, I feel confident that we can prevent him from harming himself or others under his immediate parameters of incarceration where he is in an individual room with limited access to anything that he could harm himself with or harm anyone else with, and he remains under constant observation." The panel concluded that involuntary medication was not "essential" for safety and instructed the district court that "if the government advances the medical/safety justification on remand, it will need to present additional evidence showing that either Weston's condition or his confinement

---

4 Defense counsel also claims that Weston's decision while he was medically competent not to take antipsychotic medication makes such medication medically inappropriate. We shall assume *arguendo* [for the sake of argument] that Weston's previous decision reflects his current informed judgment (which of course is unknowable). Nonetheless, withholding of consent does not make a treatment medically inappropriate. In *Harper*, for instance, the inmate reportedly said he "would rather die than take medication," but the Court approved the treatment as in the inmate's medical interest.

situation has changed since the hearing so as to render him dangerous."

In *Riggins*, the Court prescribed the conditions sufficient for a dangerousness justification, but explicitly declined to "prescribe substantive standards" for determining when other government interests override a pretrial detainee's liberty interest in refusing antipsychotic medication. The Court did, however, suggest that the governmental interest in restoring a pretrial detainee's competence to stand trial could override his liberty interest: "The State might have been able to justify medically appropriate, involuntary treatment with [antipsychotic medication] by establishing that it could not obtain an adjudication of [the pretrial detainee's] guilt or innocence by using less intrusive means."

Preventing and punishing criminality are essential governmental policies. We need not decide under what circumstances trying and punishing offenders is not "essential." The government's interest in finding, convicting, and punishing criminals reaches its zenith when the crime is the murder of federal police officers in a place crowded with bystanders where a branch of government conducts its business. The statutory sentences for the crimes Weston is accused of committing - life in prison and death - reflect the intensity of the government's interest in bringing those suspected of such crimes to trial. Weston concedes that in "the ordinary case, the strength of the government's interest in trying a defendant accused of first degree murder is undisputed," but argues that when "the government seeks to forcibly medicate a defendant in order to try him, however, the case is no longer ordinary, because presumptions against forced medication have deep roots in the law." The "presumption" against forced medication goes to the importance of Weston's constitutional right to refuse antipsychotic drugs (which we agree is substantial), not to the nature of the government's countervailing interest.

We also do not believe that the "governmental interest in medicating a defendant in order to try him is diminished by the option of civil commitment." The civil commitment argument assumes that the government's essential penological interests lie only in incapacitating dangerous offenders. It ignores the retributive, deterrent, communicative, and investigative functions of the criminal justice system, which serve to ensure that offenders receive their just desserts, to make clear that offenses entail consequences, and to discover what happened through the public mechanism of trial. Civil commitment addresses none of these interests. In Weston's case, civil commitment would be based on his present mental condition, not on his culpability for the crimes charged: "Criminal responsibility at the time of the alleged offenses is a distinct issue from his competency to stand trial."

The sole constitutional mechanism for the government to accomplish its essential policy is to take Weston to trial. Antipsychotic medication is necessary because, as the district court found, "Antipsychotic medication is the only therapeutic intervention available that could possibly improve Weston's symptom picture, lessen his delusions, and make him competent to stand trial." The government cannot "obtain an adjudication of [Weston's] guilt or innocence by using less intrusive means" (*Riggins*).

The government has established a sufficient likelihood that antipsychotic medication will restore Weston's competence while preserving his right to a fair trial. The small possibility that antipsychotic medication will not make Weston competent for trial is certainly tolerable considering that antipsychotic medication is the sole means for the government to satisfy its essential policy in adjudicating the murder of federal officers. The district court made the most precise predictive judgment it could in this context. Weston points out that there is also a possibility that antipsychotic medication could prejudice his right to a fair trial by, for instance, altering his courtroom demeanor, interfering with his recollection and ability to testify, and obstructing his right to present an insanity defense. We agree with the district court that "there is no reason to conclude, at this time, that involuntary medication would preclude Weston from receiving a fair trial."

The general right to a fair trial includes several specific rights such as the right to be tried only while competent, that is, while able to understand the proceedings, consult with counsel, and assist in the defense. As we determined, there is a sufficiently high probability that antipsychotic medication will restore Weston's competence to stand

> **There is no reason to conclude, at this time, that involuntary medication would preclude Weston from receiving a fair trial.**

trial. The district court found and the evidence indicates that "a strong likelihood exists that medication will enhance some of Weston's trial rights, particularly his right to consult with counsel and to assist in his defense."

Another aspect of the right to a fair trial is Weston's right to testify and "to present his own version of events in his own words" (*Rock v. Arkansas*). The defense is concerned that the medication might affect Weston's memory and his capacity to relate his delusions and other aspects of his mental state at the time of the crime, which in turn "may impair his ability to mount an effective insanity defense." But the record contains no basis to suppose that antipsychotic drugs will prevent Weston from testifying in a meaningful way. Rather, it indicates that medication will more likely improve Weston's ability to relate his belief system to the jury. The benefits of antipsychotic medication in terms of Weston's ability to understand the proceedings and communicate with his attorneys presumably will also translate into an improved capacity to communicate from the witness stand. And although memory loss is a potential side effect, Dr. Johnson testified that she thought "he'd be able to remember his belief system."

There is a possibility that the medication could affect Weston's behavior and demeanor on the witness stand such that the jury might regard his "synthetically sane" testimony as inconsistent with a claim of insanity. As Justice Kennedy put it in *Riggins*, "If the defendant takes the stand his demeanor can have a great bearing on his credibility and persuasiveness, and on the degree to which he evokes sympathy." We recognize this small risk, but we see little basis to suppose that the jury will take Weston's testimony (if he decides to testify) as an indication that he must have been sane at the time of the crime, or that he is making it up, or that he deserves no sympathy. There is ample evidence of Weston's history of mental illness and bizarre behavior; the jury's overall impression of Weston will depend as much on this evidence as his testimony.

The district court also correctly held that a defendant does not have an absolute right to replicate on the witness stand his mental state at the time of the crime. A defendant asserting a heat-of-passion defense to a charge of first-degree murder does not have the right to whip up a frenzy in court to show his capacity for rage, nor does a defendant claiming intoxication have the right to testify under the influence. There is little meaningful distinction between these cases and medication-induced competence to stand trial. Either way, the defendant's mental state on the stand is different from the mental state he claims to have operated under at the time of the crime. The tolerable level of difference no doubt increases in a case like this where there is substantial evidence of mental state other than the defendant's present appearance.

> *A defendant asserting a heat-of-passion defense to a charge of first-degree murder does not have the right to whip up a frenzy in court to show his capacity for rage, nor does a defendant claiming intoxication have the right to testify under the influence.*

Weston will not have to rely solely on his own testimony to show his state of mind on July 24, 1998. Involuntary medication therefore stands little chance of impairing his right to present an insanity defense. There is extensive documentation and testimony concerning Weston's delusional system, his history of mental illness, and his "behavior, appearance, speech, actions, and extraordinary or bizarre acts over a significant period." Multiple experts have examined Weston and presumably may testify. Many of these examinations no doubt related to his trial competence, but "the tapes and psychiatric reports document Weston's delusional state over several years." There is also a taped interview in which Weston discussed his delusional beliefs with the Central Intelligence Agency. Given the wealth of expert and lay testimony and other documentation the district court described, Weston's insanity defense does not stand or fall on his testimony alone.

A third trial right that could be implicated by antipsychotic medication is Weston's right to be present at trial in a state that does not prejudice the factfinder against him. To the extent the medication alters Weston's demeanor, courtroom behavior, or reactions to events in the courtroom, it may cause the jury to see Weston in a state that might seem inconsistent with a claim of insanity. It could also produce a flattened emotional affect that could convey to the jury a lack of remorse, a critical consideration if this case proceeded to sentencing.

Here again the record indicates that medication will likely enhance rather than impair Weston's right to a fair trial. Dr. Johnson stated that medication "will alter Weston's demeanor to the extent that it will be more a return to his baseline nonpsychotic state. I would anticipate he would have less blunting or flattening of his affect. He would be able to respond more appropriately from an emotional standpoint with his facial expression than he is now." The possibility of side effects from antipsychotic medication is undeniable, but the ability of Weston's treating physicians and the district court to respond to them substantially reduces the risk they pose to trial fairness. The district court found that Weston's doctors can manage side effects in a number of ways: "The Court credits the testimony of the government experts and Dr. Daniel, the independent expert, that the side effects of medication are manageable through adjustments in the timing and amount of the doses, and through supplementary medications." As the Court

> *Antipsychotic drugs have progressed since Justice Kennedy discussed their side effects in Riggins.*

wrote in *Harper*, the "risks associated with antipsychotic drugs are for the most part medical ones, best assessed by medical professionals."[5]

The district court also has measures at its disposal: "If Weston is medicated and his competency is restored, the Court is willing to take whatever reasonable measures are necessary to ensure that his rights are protected. This may include informing the jurors that Weston is being administered mind-altering medication, that his behavior in their presence is conditioned on drugs being administered to him at the request of the government, and allowing experts and others to testify regarding Weston's unmedicated condition, the effects of the medication on Weston, and the necessity of medication to render Weston competent to stand trial." Weston is free to propose other options.

There is a very high probability that involuntary medication will serve the government's essential interest in rendering Weston "competent to stand trial in a proceeding that is fair to both parties" (*United States v. Brandon*). Given the lack of alternative means for the government to satisfy its essential policy, we cannot demand more. Because antipsychotic medication is medically appropriate and is necessary to accomplish an essential state policy, the district court's order permitting the government to forcibly medicate Weston is affirmed.

---

[5] Antipsychotic drugs have progressed since Justice Kennedy discussed their side effects in *Riggins*. There is a new generation of medications having better side effect profiles. Although the government presently plans to medicate Weston with the older generation of typicals, it could switch to the newer atypicals if side effects from the typicals threaten to impair his right to a fair trial.

United States v. Brandon

158 F.3d 947 (6th Circuit, 1998)

Facts

In 1996, Ralph Brandon was charged with sending threatening communications through the mail. He was evaluated at the Federal Medical Center (FMC) Lexington, Kentucky, and diagnosed with paranoid schizophrenia. He was found incompetent and sent to FMC Rochester, Minnesota, for competency restoration treatment. The district court instructed FMC Rochester that Brandon was not to be involuntarily administered antipsychotic medication without the district court's approval. Staff recommended that he be medicated as the least restrictive means available to restore competency. Brandon argued that an evidentiary hearing was required. The court disagreed and indicated an internal administrative hearing was adequate to protect his rights.

Under Bureau Of Prisons (BOP) procedures set forth in the Code of Federal Regulations, an individual committed to the custody of the Attorney General, such as Brandon, is afforded an administrative hearing before he or she may be forcibly medicated with psychotropic medication. Such individuals are provided the following procedural safeguards:

- 24-hour written notice of the time, date, place, and purpose of the hearing, with the reasons for the proposed medication.
- Notice of the right to appear, present evidence, and be represented by a staff member at the hearing.
- The hearing is conducted by a psychiatrist not currently involved in the diagnosis or treatment of the individual.
- The mental health professional treating or evaluating the individual must attend the hearing and present clinical data and background information in support of the need for medication.
- The psychiatrist conducting the hearing determines and prepares a written report regarding the necessity of such medication (i.e., whether such medication is necessary in the effort to restore the individual's competence, or because

the individual is dangerous, gravely disabled, or unable to function in his housing facility).

- The individual is given a copy of the report and notified of the right to appeal the determination to the administrator of the mental health division of the institution within 24 hours of the decision.
- No medication is administered until resolution of the appeal.
- A nonattending psychiatrist must monitor the individual's treatment at least once every 30 days and document the same.
- Only in emergency situations may an individual be medicated prior to a hearing or while an appeal is pending. During an emergency, an individual may be forcibly medicated only when doing so is an "appropriate treatment" and no less restrictive means are available.

Brandon claimed that constitutional due process required the forced-medication decision to be made in the context of a judicial hearing with additional procedural safeguards not provided for by BOP regulations. The government contended that an administrative hearing pursuant to BOP regulations sufficiently protected Brandon's due process rights.

Issue

Does the Due Process Clause of the Fifth Amendment require a judicial hearing to determine whether a nondangerous pretrial detainee can be forcibly medicated in order to attempt to render him competent to stand trial? Does an administrative hearing in accord with BOP regulations provide sufficient procedural safeguards for the nondangerous pretrial detainee when determining whether involuntary medication is authorized?

Holding

Due process considerations require a judicial hearing on the issue of whether a nondangerous pretrial detainee may be forcibly medicated in order to render him competent to stand trial. The BOP regulations do not provide sufficient procedural safeguards for the nondangerous pretrial detainee when determining whether involuntary medication is authorized.

Analysis

Four factors were considered. The first among these were the interests of the private individual. In considering these, the court endorsed questionable views that psychiatric medication is inherently detrimental or risky, including (1) medication might diminish defendants' capacity to communicate ideas, (2) medication side effects can be severe and irreversible, (3) medication might create a "prejudicial negative demeanor," and (4) medication might impair ability to assist counsel. The second factor was the government's legitimate interest in seeking convictions. The constitutional power to bring an accused to trial is fundamental to "ordered liberty and a prerequisite to social justice and peace." Third, the court weighed the value of a judicial hearing. This case differed from *Washington v. Harper* and *Parham v. J.R.*, which both held that medical professionals are better qualified than judges to make medical decisions, where issues were strictly medical in nature. In *Brandon*, the primary issue - competency - is judicial rather than medical. The burden of attending a judicial hearing was not viewed as "overbearing in light of the weightiness" of this issue. Fourth, the risks of an administrative hearing were analyzed. The court concluded that since *Brandon* involved legal issues, and psychologists and psychiatrists have no legal training, the decision requires an evidentiary hearing.

Edited Excerpts[1]

United States of America, Plaintiff-Appellee v. Ralph E. Brandon, Defendant-Appellant

United States Court of Appeals Sixth Circuit

158 F.3d 947

October 23, 1998

Before: Keith, Ryan, and Gilman, Circuit Judges

Gilman, Circuit Judge

Ralph E. Brandon, currently in jail awaiting trial on the criminal charge of sending a threatening letter through the mail,

---

[1] Readers are advised to quote only from the original published cases. See pages vii-viii.

appeals from the district court's order denying him a judicial hearing on the issue of whether he may be forcibly medicated with antipsychotic drugs in order to render him competent to stand trial. The government asserts that Brandon's interlocutory appeal is premature and lacking in merit. For the reasons that follow, we find that appellate review is appropriate and hold that Brandon is entitled to a judicial hearing to decide whether he may be forcibly medicated. We therefore reverse the district court's ruling and remand the case for further proceedings consistent with this opinion.

On October 1, 1996, Brandon was indicted on the charge of sending a threatening communication to a "C. Bailey" through the mail. Brandon's attorney moved for a court-ordered competency evaluation. On November 20, 1996, the district court granted the motion and placed Brandon in the custody of the Attorney General for a psychiatric examination to determine whether Brandon was competent to stand trial. An evaluation was conducted in February of 1997 by the Federal Medical Center in Lexington, Kentucky (FMC Lexington). A forensic psychologist at FMC Lexington diagnosed Brandon as a paranoid schizophrenic,

The issue on appeal is whether a BOP administrative hearing provides sufficient due process to determine whether antipsychotic medication can be forcibly administered to Brandon in order to render him competent to stand trial.

and concluded that he is "mentally incompetent to the extent that he is unable to understand the nature and consequences of proceedings against him or to assist properly in his defense."

On March 4, 1997, the district court held a competency hearing. Based on the psychiatric evaluation report and the agreement of counsel, the district court concluded that Brandon was not competent to stand trial. The district court then committed Brandon to the Federal Medical Center in Rochester, Minnesota (FMC Rochester) for a determination of whether there was "a substantial probability that in the foreseeable future defendant will attain the capacity to permit the trial to proceed." The district court instructed the Bureau of Prison's (BOP) hospital at FMC Rochester that it could not involuntarily administer Brandon antipsychotic medication without the approval of the district court. On April 9, 1997, FMC Rochester sent the district court an Admission Psychiatric Evaluation Addendum (APEA), recommending that Brandon be given antipsychotic medication, which Brandon had refused to take. The APEA concluded as follows:

"His multidisciplinary team concurs with the diagnosis of Delusional Disorder and the need for antipsychotic medication as the least restrictive alternative to restore him to competency." FMC Rochester further reminded the district court that the medication would be administered only after the hospital held an administrative hearing and upon direction from the district court.

Brandon then moved for an evidentiary hearing to determine whether the hospital could force him to take antipsychotic medication. The district court denied the motion on July 18, 1997, holding that an administrative hearing conducted by the hospital on the medication issue would suffice to protect Brandon's due process rights. Brandon thereafter appealed from the district court's order, and filed an emergency application for a stay pending the appeal. On July 31, 1997, this court issued an order refusing to stay the district court's order to the extent that it allowed the BOP's administrative hearing to proceed, but granted a stay that prohibited the administration of antipsychotic medication without prior approval by this court. On November 4, 1997, FMC Rochester's Warden sent a letter to the district court reporting that an administrative hearing was conducted on July 30, 1997. The hearing officer concluded that Brandon should be forcibly medicated with antipsychotic drugs.

Brandon's appeal presents whether the Due Process Clause of the Fifth Amendment[2] requires a judicial hearing to determine whether a nondangerous pretrial detainee can be forcibly medicated in order to render him competent to stand trial. Whether Brandon may be forcibly medicated, however, is not the issue presently on appeal. The issue on appeal is whether a BOP administrative hearing provides sufficient due process to determine whether antipsychotic medication can be forcibly administered to Brandon in order to render him competent to stand trial. The issue to be determined is what procedural safeguards must be provided in a hearing to make that decision. The district court has conclusively decided that a BOP administrative

> **Brandon claims that his constitutional due process rights require that the forced-medication decision be made in the context of a judicial hearing.**

hearing will satisfy due process requirements and that a judicial hearing is not required. This issue has therefore been conclusively decided by the district court.

---

[2] Fifth Amendment. See Appendix B (p. 261).

In 1979, the Supreme Court issued its decision in *Parham v. J.R.*, holding that Georgia's mental-health laws regarding involuntary civil commitment proceedings provided sufficient procedural safeguards for minors. The Court weighed the child's substantial liberty interest in avoiding unnecessary confinement against the state's *parens patriae* interest in protecting the welfare of the child. (*Parens patriae*, literally "parent of the country," refers traditionally to the role of the state as sovereign and guardian of persons under legal disability, such as juveniles or the insane.) The Court rejected the need for a judicial hearing on what it held was essentially a medical decision. The Court explained that minors are best protected when decisions regarding their best interests are reserved to medical professionals, rather than to a judge. The Court reasserted its deference to medical judgment in *Youngberg v. Romeo*, holding that a mental health facility could exercise its *parens patriae* power to physically restrain an incompetent inmate, so long as the decision was made within the exercise of professional medical judgment.

The Tenth Circuit, in *Bee v. Greaves*, held that the forced medication of a pretrial detainee would affect the detainee's ability to produce ideas and, therefore, affected the detainee's freedom of speech. While the court noted that Bee was eventually found competent, it questioned whether bringing him to trial could ever be a sufficiently compelling reason to medicate him against his will. In *United States v. Charters* (*en banc*[3]), the Fourth Circuit extended the "medical judgment" standard in deciding whether to forcibly medicate a dangerous pretrial detainee. The court relied on *Parham* and *Youngberg*, holding that a judicial hearing was not necessary or valuable for making the "baseline" determination, but such a hearing should be conducted to review the hospital's decision for the purpose of ensuring that it was not arbitrary.

In *Washington v. Harper*, the Supreme Court applied this deference to medical judgment in a case involving the forced medication of a dangerous convicted felon. The government's interest at stake in *Harper* was the safety conditions within the prison. Relying on *Parham*, the Court concluded that such medical decisions were not aided by judicial intervention. The Court also applied a "rational-basis" standard of review, holding that

> **No one disputes that the government's interest in bringing a defendant to trial is substantial.**

---

[3] *en banc.* All the judges of an appellate court considering an opinion together.

the regulation was reasonably related to legitimate penological interests. In *Riggins v. Nevada*, the Supreme Court declined to prescribe substantive standards to define when a pretrial detainee awaiting trial on murder and robbery charges may be forcibly medicated. The Court described *Harper* as requiring that a decision to forcibly medicate a prisoner be based on a finding of an overriding justification for and the medical appropriateness of the treatment, and reversed the district court's order, which allowed forced medication without considering the need for such treatment or the availability of reasonable alternatives. The Supreme Court went on to say, however, that such a decision would be constitutional if based on a finding that no less restrictive alternatives were available, and that such medication was necessary for either safety reasons or to obtain a proper adjudication of guilt or innocence.

The only case decided since *Harper* and *Riggins* that discusses whether a pretrial detainee is entitled to a judicial hearing before being medicated for the purpose of restoring competency to stand trial is *Van Khiem v. United States*. Quoting *Parham*, the Van Khiem court extended the medical-judgment rule to non-dangerous pretrial detainees, holding that "due process is not violated by the use of informal traditional medical investigative techniques." The court did not offer any reason for this conclusion other than its understanding that *Parham* and *Harper* do not require adversarial proceedings.

The government argues that an administrative hearing sufficiently protects Brandon's due process rights. A determination of what procedural safeguards are required is a constitutional issue to be reviewed *de novo*.[4] We must consider the following four factors: (1) the private individual's interests, (2) the government's interests, including the fiscal and administrative burdens at stake, (3) the value of the suggested procedural requirements, and (4) the risk of erroneous deprivation of the individual's rights that is inherent in current procedures. Procedural due process rules are shaped by "the risk of error inherent in the truth-finding process as applied to the generality of cases, not the rare exceptions."

Brandon's interests in avoiding forced medication are several and significant. He has a First Amendment[5] interest in avoiding forced medication, which may interfere with his ability to communicate ideas. See *Bee v. Greaves*, "Antipsychotic drugs have the capacity to severely and even permanently affect an individual's

---

[4] *de novo*. Over again; anew.
[5] First Amendment. See Appendix B (p. 261).

ability to think and communicate." Further, the issue of forced medication implicates Brandon's Fifth Amendment[6] liberty interest in being free from bodily intrusion. As mentioned in *Harper*, the purpose of these medications is to alter the chemical balance in the patient's brain in order to restore his cognitive abilities. Although the various drugs might have beneficial results, the concomitant side effects might be severe and irreversible. For example, the court in *Harper* referred to expert testimony stating that 10% to 25% of the patients taking antipsychotic medication develop tardive dyskinesia, which is characterized by uncontrollable movements of various muscles of the body and face. Also involved is Brandon's Sixth Amendment right to a fair trial. As Justice Kennedy said in his concurring opinion in *Riggins*: "By administering medication, the State may be creating a prejudicial negative demeanor in the defendant - making him look nervous and restless, for example, or so calm or sedated as to appear bored, cold, unfeeling, and unresponsive. . . ." Justice Kennedy warned that the mind-altering effect of the medication may also impinge on a defendant's right to effective assistance of counsel by rendering him unable or unwilling to assist in the preparation of his own defense.

The government does not contend that Brandon is a danger to himself or others. Rather, the government's interest in this case is to render Brandon competent to stand trial in a proceeding that is fair to both parties. If the government fails in this effort, it must dismiss the indictment and proceed with a civil-commitment hearing. No one disputes that the government's interest in bringing a defendant to trial is substantial.

Both *Parham* and *Harper* dealt with the strictly medical issue of what treatment was in the best interests of the individuals in custody. In both cases, the treatment was held to be constitutional so long as the medical professionals considered it appropriate in the exercise of their professional judgment. But *Parham* dealt with the civil commitment of a minor and *Harper* dealt with a dangerous convicted felon. The present case, in contrast, involves a nondangerous pretrial detainee. The decision to be made here is whether the detainee may be forcibly medicated so as to render him competent to stand trial, not whether treatment with drugs is in the detainee's medical interests. This decision will require the court to consider whether the medication will have a prejudicial effect on Brandon's physical appearance at trial, as

---

[6] Fifth Amendment. See Appendix B (p. 261).

well as whether it will interfere with his ability to aid in the preparation of his own defense.

The district court will have to make difficult legal decisions after hearing all of the medical evidence. Physicians are not equipped to determine the effect that the drugs will have on Brandon's right to a fair trial and right to counsel. Rather, the district court must understand and apply the medical recommendations of the physicians in making such decisions. The district court will benefit greatly if the FMC physicians are available for elaboration and clarification of the indications and side effects of the medication. Furthermore, the burden on the testifying physicians of attending a judicial hearing is not overbearing in light of the weightiness of the decision to be made - whether to forcibly medicate a person presumed innocent in order to restore his competency to stand trial. We therefore conclude that due process considerations require a judicial hearing on the issue presented in the case before us.

Having decided that such a hearing is necessary, there is little extra burden on the government to allow Brandon to present his own rebuttal testimony on the issues involved. The drawback of this approach is that it may result in a "battle of the experts," requiring the judge to evaluate potentially inconsistent medical opinions. There is no more risk of error in allowing the consideration of several medical opinions, however, than exists in totally deferring to one such opinion. In fact, it might be especially important to allow consideration of more than one medical judgment in such cases where experts are likely to disagree. In any event, judges are frequently required to decide which expert's opinion is the most persuasive.

As previously stated, the key decisions to be made in the present case involve nonmedical issues, such as the effect the medication will have on Brandon's right to a fair trial and his right to counsel. There is obviously great risk in allowing this determination to be made at an administrative hearing by BOP physicians who have no legal training. Given the above considerations, we find that the BOP regulation does not provide

> *Physicians are not equipped to determine the effect that the drugs will have on Brandon's right to a fair trial and right to counsel.*

sufficient procedural safeguards for deciding whether to forcibly medicate a nondangerous pretrial detainee. Accordingly, we conclude that such a decision requires an evidentiary hearing, and remand this case so that such a proceeding may be conducted.

Government action subject to strict scrutiny survives only if it is narrowly tailored to a compelling governmental interest. The decision of whether the government's interest in medicating a pretrial detainee is compelling must be made in light of (1) whether the pretrial detainee is dangerous to himself or others, (2) the seriousness of the crime, and (3) whether the detainee will be released from confinement if not made to stand trial. Whether the proposed treatment is narrowly tailored to this interest will turn on whether it is the least restrictive and least harmful means of satisfying the government's goal - in this case, of rendering Brandon competent to stand trial in a proceeding that is fair to both parties. When making this determination, the district court should engage in a two-step analysis. In the first step of the analysis, the court will receive medical testimony regarding Brandon's mental illness and its symptoms, as well as the effects that antipsychotic medication will have, both beneficial and harmful, on Brandon's physical and mental health. This step involves an analysis of Brandon's condition and treatment that is essentially medical. In the second part of the analysis, the district court will then have to make the legal determination of whether Brandon, if forcibly medicated, would be competent to participate in a trial that is fair to both parties. This will require consideration of whether the medication will have a prejudicial effect on Brandon's physical appearance at trial, as well as whether it will interfere with his ability to aid in the preparation of his own defense. In particular, the district court needs to consider the risks that forced medication poses to a pretrial detainee such as Brandon, because a drug that negatively affects his demeanor in court or ability to participate in his own defense will not satisfy the government's goal of a fair trial.

This legal determination is distinct from the medical determination that the medical experts will discuss in step one of the analysis. Antipsychotic medication might sedate Brandon, making him appear to be lucid and rational, for example, but might not make him in fact lucid and rational. It is important, therefore, that the medical experts testify about the chemical and behavioral effects of the proposed medication, leaving to the district court the ultimate conclusion of whether those effects will render Brandon legally competent, that is, whether Brandon would be able to receive a fair trial if forcibly medicated.

We next address the proper burden of proof to be applied in deciding whether to forcibly medicate a nondangerous pretrial detainee. We find persuasive the case of *Addington v. Texas*. The Supreme Court in *Addington* held that in order to civilly commit an individual, the government is required to prove by clear and convincing evidence that the individual is mentally ill. The Court stated that the individual's interests involved in a civil commitment proceeding are greater than exist in a civil case concerning only monetary damages, but less than that present in a criminal case where an individual may face a wrongful conviction. The Court also explained that a higher level of proof is necessary to preserve fundamental fairness in government-initiated proceedings that threaten the individual involved with "a significant deprivation of liberty" or "stigma."

The Court stated as follows: "The individual should not be asked to share equally with society the risk of error when the possible injury to the individual is significantly greater than any possible harm to the state. We conclude that the individual's interest in the outcome of a civil commitment proceeding is of such weight and gravity that due process requires the state to justify confinement by proof more substantial than a mere preponderance of the evidence." We believe that the risk of error and possible harm involved in deciding whether to forcibly medicate an incompetent, nondangerous pretrial detainee are likewise so substantial as to require the government to prove its case by clear and convincing evidence. Given the current risks associated with the administration of antipsychotic medication, no other standard would sufficiently protect Brandon's rights.

Although the ultimate decision must be made by the district court on remand, we fully recognize the difficult burden faced by the government on this issue. But this is as it should be, given the interests at stake. The government correctly argues that it has a "significant" interest in prosecuting Brandon, rather than having to pursue civil commitment proceedings. We find it difficult to imagine, however, that the government's interest in prosecuting the charge of sending a threatening letter through the mail could be considered a compelling justification to forcibly medicate Brandon. This case involves no safety concerns, because Brandon has not been deemed to be dangerous. Further, the maximum penalty for sending a threatening communication is five years imprisonment. As Justice Kennedy, who authored the Court's opinion in *Harper*, wrote in *Riggins*: "Absent an extraordinary showing by the State, the Due Process

> **We find it difficult to imagine that the government's interest in prosecuting the charge of sending a threatening letter through the mail could be considered a compelling justification to forcibly medicate Brandon.**

Clause prohibits prosecuting officials from administering involuntary doses of antipsychotic medicines for purposes of rendering the accused competent to stand trial, and express doubt that the showing can be made in most cases, given our present understanding of the properties of these drugs."

We agree with this position. Although this higher burden of proof was rejected in *Harper*, it was done in a context inapposite to the present case. In *Harper*, the Supreme Court held that the decision to medicate a dangerous convicted felon could be made solely by medical professionals without the need for a judicial hearing. Based on that fact, the Court concluded it would make no sense to require medical professionals to convince themselves of the medical appropriateness of their own decision by clear and convincing evidence. Here, however, we are dealing with a non-dangerous pretrial detainee, where a judge must conduct an evidentiary hearing on the forced-medication issue for all of the reasons previously discussed. Therefore, *Harper*'s reasoning does not apply to the facts of this case.

For all of the reasons stated above, we reverse the district court's ruling and remand the case for further proceedings consistent with this opinion. The emergency stay granted by this court against forcibly medicating Brandon shall remain in effect until the final resolution of this case.

Sell v. United States

539 U.S. ___ (U.S. Supreme Court, 2003)[1]

Facts

A dentist from an affluent St. Louis suburb, Charles Sell, was charged with numerous counts of insurance and mail fraud in 1995. He was later charged with conspiring to kill witnesses, including an FBI agent. Following an involuntary medication hearing like that described in *Brandon*, a psychiatrist authorized treatment with antipsychotic medications against the defendant's will. Defense counsel appealed this decision directly to the courts, where it was upheld at the level of the U.S. Magistrate Judge, who authorized involuntary medication on the basis of both competency restoration and the defendant's dangerousness. The U.S. District Court reversed the ruling that Sell was dangerous, noting that he was not dangerous in the "institutional context" of a federal medical center, and upheld the involuntary medication decision solely on the basis of competency restoration. The 8th Circuit Court of Appeals affirmed.

Issue

Does the Constitution permit the government to administer antipsychotic medications to a mentally ill criminal defendant on an involuntary basis solely to restore the defendant to competency to stand trial? The Supreme Court accepted a narrow question, limited to nondangerous pretrial detainees.

Holding

The Constitution does permit such involuntary medication in limited circumstances.

Analysis

Involuntary medication of nondangerous defendants is permissible only when "important governmental interests are at stake." Additionally, the court ordering involuntary application of medica-

---

[1] This is a preliminary, unpublished opinion by the Supreme Court (a "slip opinion") and the ultimate citation has yet to be determined.

tion for the sole purpose of restoring competency to stand trial must find (1) the medications are "substantially likely" to render the defendant competent, (2) the treatment will not "interfere significantly with the defendant's ability to assist counsel in conducting a trial defense, thereby rendering the trial unfair," (3) "alternative, less intrusive treatments" are unlikely to restore competency, and (4) the treatment must be "medically appropriate." Clinicians retain the authority to administer medication on an involuntary basis for other purposes, such as treatment of grave disability or attempts to reduce or prevent dangerous behavior, as described in *Harper* or *Riggins*. In such instances, the judicial inquiry described in *Sell* is unnecessary.

Edited Excerpts[2]

Sell v. United States

Certiorari to the 8th Circuit Court of Appeals

Supreme Court of the United States

539 U.S. ___

June 16, 2003

Justice Breyer delivered the opinion of the Court, in which Rehnquist, C.J., and Stevens, Kennedy, Souter, and Ginsburg, JJ., joined. Scalia, J. filed a dissenting opinion, in which O'Connor and Thomas, JJ. Joined.

The question presented is whether the Constitution permits the Government to administer antipsychotic drugs involuntarily to a mentally ill criminal defendant - in order to render that defendant competent to stand trial for serious, but nonviolent, crimes. We conclude that the Constitution allows the Government to administer those drugs, even against the defendant's will, in limited circumstances, that is, upon satisfaction of conditions that we shall describe. Because the Court of Appeals did not find that the requisite circumstances existed in this case, we vacate its judgment.

---

[2] Readers are advised to quote only from the original published cases. See pages vii-viii.

Petitioner Charles Sell, once a practicing dentist, has a long and unfortunate history of mental illness. In September 1982, after telling doctors that the gold he used for fillings had been contaminated by communists, Sell was hospitalized, treated with antipsychotic medication, and subsequently discharged. In June 1984, Sell called the police to say that a leopard was outside his office boarding a bus, and he then asked the police to shoot him. Sell was again hospitalized and subsequently released. On various occasions, he complained that public officials were trying to kill him. In April 1997, he told law enforcement personnel that he "spoke to God last night," and that "God told me every [Federal Bureau of Investigation] person I kill, a soul will be saved."

In May 1997, the Government charged Sell with submitting fictitious insurance claims for payment. A Federal Magistrate Judge (Magistrate), after ordering a psychiatric examination, found Sell "currently competent," but noted that Sell might experience "a psychotic episode" in the future. The judge released Sell on bail. A grand jury later produced a superseding indictment charging Sell and his wife with 56 counts of mail fraud, 6 counts of Medicaid fraud, and 1 count of money laundering.

> **Does forced administration of antipsychotic drugs to render Sell competent to stand trial unconstitutionally deprive him of his "liberty" to reject medical treatment?**

In early 1998, the Government claimed that Sell had sought to intimidate a witness. The Magistrate held a bail revocation hearing. Sell's behavior at his initial appearance was, in the judge's words, "totally out of control," involving "screaming and shouting," the use of "personal insults" and "racial epithets," and spitting "in the judge's face." A psychiatrist reported that Sell could not sleep because he expected the FBI to "come busting through the door," and concluded that Sell's condition had worsened. After considering that report and other testimony, the Magistrate revoked Sell's bail.

In April 1998, the grand jury issued a new indictment charging Sell with attempting to murder the FBI agent who had arrested him and a former employee who planned to testify against him in the fraud case. The attempted murder and fraud cases were joined for trial. In early 1999, Sell asked the Magistrate to reconsider his competence to stand trial. The Magistrate sent Sell to the United States Medical Center for Federal Prisoners at Springfield, Missouri, for examination. Subsequently the Magistrate found that Sell was "mentally incompetent to stand trial." He ordered Sell to "be

> **A court must find that important governmental interests are at stake.**

hospitalized for treatment" at the Medical Center for up to four months, "to determine whether there was a substantial probability that Sell would attain the capacity to allow his trial to proceed." Two months later, Medical Center staff recommended that Sell take antipsychotic medication. Sell refused to do so. The staff sought permission to administer the medication against Sell's will. That effort is the subject of the present proceedings.

We turn now to the basic question presented: Does forced administration of antipsychotic drugs to render Sell competent to stand trial unconstitutionally deprive him of his "liberty" to reject medical treatment?

Two prior precedents, *Harper* and *Riggins*, set forth the framework for determining the legal answer. These two cases indicate that the Constitution permits the Government involuntarily to administer antipsychotic drugs to a mentally ill defendant facing serious criminal charges in order to render that defendant competent to stand trial, but only if the treatment is medically appropriate, is substantially unlikely to have side effects that may undermine the fairness of the trial, and, taking account of less intrusive alternatives, is necessary significantly to further important governmental trial-related interests.

This standard will permit involuntary administration of drugs solely for trial competence purposes in certain instances. But those instances may be rare. That is because the standard says or fairly implies the following.

First, a court must find that *important* governmental interests are at stake. The Government's interest in bringing to trial an individual accused of a serious crime is important. That is so whether the offense is a serious crime against the person or a serious crime against property. In both instances the Government seeks to protect through application of the criminal law the basic human need for security. Courts, however, must consider the facts of the individual case in evaluating the Government's interest in prosecution. Special circumstances may lessen the importance of that interest. The defendant's failure to take drugs voluntarily, for example, may mean lengthy confinement in an institution for the mentally ill - and that would diminish the risks that ordinarily attach to freeing without punishment one who has committed a serious crime. We do not mean

> **The Government has a substantial interest in timely prosecution. The Government has a concomitant, constitutionally essential interest in assuring that the defendant's trial is a fair one.**

to suggest that civil commitment is a substitute for a criminal trial. The Government has a substantial interest in timely prosecution.

And it may be difficult or impossible to try a defendant who regains competence after years of commitment during which memories may fade and evidence may be lost. The potential for future confinement affects, but does not totally undermine, the strength of the need for prosecution. The same is true of the possibility that the defendant has already been confined for a significant amount of time (for which he would receive credit toward any sentence ultimately imposed). Moreover, the Government has a concomitant, constitutionally essential interest in assuring that the defendant's trial is a fair one.

Second, the court must conclude that involuntary medication will *significantly further* those concomitant state interests. It must find that administration of the drugs is substantially likely to render the defendant competent to stand trial. At the same time, it must find that administration of the drugs is substantially unlikely to have side effects that will interfere significantly with the defendant's ability to assist counsel in conducting a trial defense, thereby rendering the trial unfair.

Third, the court must conclude that involuntary medication is *necessary* to further those interests. The court must find that any alternative, less intrusive treatments are unlikely to achieve substantially the same results. And the court must consider less intrusive means for admin-

> *The court must find that any alternative, less intrusive treatments are unlikely to achieve substantially the same results.*

istering the drugs, for example, a court order to the defendant backed by the contempt power, before considering more intrusive methods.

Fourth, as we have said, the court must conclude that administration of the drugs is *medically appropriate*, that is, in the patient's best medical interest in light of his medical condition. The specific kinds of drugs at issue may matter here as elsewhere. Different kinds of antipsychotic drugs may produce different side effects and enjoy different levels of success.

We emphasize that the court applying these standards is seeking to determine whether involuntary administration of drugs is necessary significantly to further a particular governmental interest, namely, the interest in rendering the defendant *competent to stand trial*. A court need not consider whether to allow forced medication for that kind of purpose, if forced medication is warranted for a *different* purpose, such as the purposes set out in *Harper* related to the individual's dangerousness, or purposes related to the individual's own interests where refusal to take drugs puts his health gravely at risk. There are often strong reasons for a court to determine whether forced administration of drugs can be justified on these alternative grounds *before* turning to the trial competence question.

For one thing, the inquiry into whether medication is permissible, say, to render an individual nondangerous is usually more "objective and manageable" than the inquiry into whether medication is permissible to render a defendant competent. The medical experts may find it easier to provide an informed opinion about whether, given the risk of side effects, particular drugs are medically appropriate and necessary to control a patient's potentially dangerous behavior (or to avoid serious harm to the patient himself) than to try to balance harms and benefits related to the more quintessentially legal questions of trial fairness and competence.

> The inquiry into whether medication is permissible to render an individual nondangerous is usually more "objective and manageable" than the inquiry into whether medication is permissible to render a defendant competent.

For another thing, courts typically address involuntary medical treatment as a civil matter, and justify it on these alternative, *Harper*-type grounds. Every State provides avenues through which, for example, a doctor or institution can seek appointment of a guardian with the power to make a decision authorizing medication - when in the best interests of a patient who lacks the mental competence to make such a decision. And courts, in civil proceedings, may authorize involuntary medication where the patient's failure to accept treatment threatens injury to the patient or others.

If a court authorizes medication on these alternative grounds, the need to consider authorization on trial competence grounds will likely disappear. Even if a court decides medication cannot be authorized on the alternative grounds, the findings underlying such a decision will help to inform expert opinion and judicial decision making in respect to a request to administer drugs for trial competence purposes. At the least, they will facilitate direct medical and legal focus upon such questions as: Why is it medically appropriate forcibly to administer antipsychotic drugs to an individual who (1) is *not* dangerous *and* (2) *is* competent to make up his own mind about treatment? Can bringing such an individual

> We consequently believe that a court, asked to approve forced administration of drugs for purposes of rendering a defendant competent to stand trial, should ordinarily determine whether the Government has first sought permission for forced administration of drugs on other grounds; and, if not, why not.

to trial *alone* justify in whole (or at least in significant part) administration of a drug that may have adverse side effects, including side
effects that may to some extent impair a defense at trial? We consequently believe that a court, asked to approve forced administration
of drugs for purposes of rendering a defendant competent to stand
trial, should ordinarily determine whether the Government seeks, or
has first sought, permission for forced administration of drugs on
these other *Harper*-type grounds; and, if not, why not.

When a court must nonetheless reach the trial competence question, the factors discussed above, should help it make the ultimate
constitutionally required judgment. Has the Government, in light of
the efficacy, the side effects, the possible alternatives, and the medical appropriateness of a particular course of antipsychotic drug
treatment, shown a need for that treatment sufficiently important to
overcome the individual's protected interest in refusing it?

Justice Scalia, With Whom O'Connor and Thomas, JJ., Join, Dissenting

The District Court never entered a final judgment in this case,
which should have led the Court of Appeals to wonder whether it
had any business entertaining petitioner's appeal. Instead, without
so much as acknowledging that Congress has limited court-of-
appeals jurisdiction to "appeals from all *final decisions* of the district
courts of the United States" (emphasis added), and appeals from certain specified interlocutory orders, the Court of Appeals proceeded to
the merits of Sell's interlocutory appeal.

The Government possessed the requisite authority to administer
forced medication. Petitioner responded, not by appealing to the
courts administrative determination, but by moving in the District
Court overseeing his criminal prosecution for a *hearing* regarding
the appropriateness of his medication.

Today's narrow holding will allow criminal defendants in petitioner's position to engage in opportunistic behavior. They can, for
example, voluntarily take
their medication until
halfway through trial, then
abruptly refuse and de-
mand an interlocutory
appeal from the order that
medication continue on a
compulsory basis. This sort

> **Today's holding will allow criminal
> defendants to voluntarily take their
> medication until halfway through
> trial, then abruptly refuse and de-
> mand an order that medication
> continue on a compulsory basis.**

of concern for the disruption of criminal proceedings - strangely
missing from the Court's discussion today - is what has led us to

state many times that we interpret the collateral-order exception narrowly in criminal cases.

But the adverse effects of today's narrow holding are as nothing compared to the adverse effects of the new rule of law that underlies the holding. The Court's opinion announces that appellate jurisdiction is proper because review after conviction and sentence will come only after "Sell will have undergone forced medication - the very harm that he seeks to avoid." This analysis effects a breathtaking expansion of appellate jurisdiction over interlocutory orders. If it is applied faithfully (and some appellate panels will be eager to apply it faithfully), any criminal defendant who asserts that a trial court order will, if implemented, cause an immediate violation of his constitutional (or perhaps even statutory?) rights may immediately appeal. He is empowered to hold up the trial for months by claiming that review after final judgment "would come too late" to prevent the violation. A trial-court order requiring the defendant to wear an electronic bracelet could be attacked as an immediate infringement of the constitutional right to "bodily integrity"; an order refusing to allow the defendant to wear a T-shirt that says "Black Power" in front of the jury could be attacked as an immediate violation of First Amendment rights; and an order compelling testimony could be attacked as an immediate denial of Fifth Amendment rights. All these orders would be immediately appealable.

Petitioner's mistaken litigation strategy, and this Court's desire to decide an interesting constitutional issue, do not justify a disregard of the limits that Congress has imposed on courts of appeals' (and our own) jurisdiction. We should vacate the judgment here, and remand the case to the Court of Appeals with instructions to dismiss.

Jackson v. Indiana

406 U.S. 715 (1972)

Facts

Theon Jackson was arrested in 1968 for two robberies, amounting to a total loss of nine dollars. Jackson was deaf, mute, and had "the mental level of a preschool child." Two evaluations determined that he would never be sufficiently competent to stand trial. The evaluations concluded he would be incompetent even if he were not deaf and mute. His intellectual abilities were not sufficient for him to acquire necessary communication skills, and Indiana had no facilities to adequately treat him. The trial court ordered Jackson confined until he was competent to proceed.

Procedural History

Jackson's counsel appealed this order to the Supreme Court of Indiana. Counsel argued that Jackson's "commitment under these circumstances amounted to a 'life sentence' without his ever having been convicted of a crime." Jackson's counsel further contended such a commitment violated Jackson's Fourteenth Amendment[1] rights to due process and equal protection, and constituted cruel and unusual punishment in violation of the Eighth Amendment.[2] If Jackson were not facing criminal charges, it was noted, he might be subjected to civil commitment proceedings which would have afforded him substantially greater rights. Despite those arguments, the Supreme Court of Indiana affirmed the trial court decision. The case was appealed to the United States Supreme Court.

---

[1] Due Process Clause of the Fourteenth Amendment (Section 1). See Appendix B (p. 262).

[2] Eighth Amendment. See Appendix B (p. 262).

Issue

Is the indefinite commitment of an incompetent defendant for the purpose of competency restoration constitutional, or does it violate the guarantees of due process and equal protection?

Holding

The Supreme Court reversed the decision, holding that it was unconstitutional to commit Jackson indefinitely. There must be a reasonable relationship between the purposes of the commitment and the duration of the commitment. In Jackson's case, civil commitment was deemed the appropriate vehicle for any necessary long-term hospitalization.

Analysis

The decision was reversed for three main reasons. First, the state should have invoked civil commitment proceedings. Standards for release of a civilly committed person are adequate to serve the interests of society because the committed individual remains under the court's control and because any release can be revoked after a hearing. Second, under civil commitment statutes, a different commitment standard would have applied, conditions of release would have been more lenient, and Jackson would have been afforded care and privileges not available in the criminal justice system. Third, Indiana law violated the Fourteenth Amendment for similar reasons. Under *Greenwood v. United States*, a person committed beyond the end of his sentence "must be released when he is no longer dangerous."

The decision emphasized a "rule of reason." The court held, "Without a finding of dangerousness, one committed can be held only for a 'reasonable period of time' necessary to determine whether there is a substantial chance of his attaining the capacity to stand trial in the foreseeable future." Furthermore, "even if it is determined that the defendant probably soon will be able to stand trial, his continued commitment must be justified by progress toward that goal."

Edited Excerpts[3]

Jackson v. Indiana

Certiorari to the Supreme Court of Indiana

Supreme Court of the United States

406 U.S. 715

June 7, 1972

Blackmun, J., delivered the opinion of the Court, in which all Members joined except Powell and Rehnquist, JJ., who took no part in the consideration or decision of the case.

We are here concerned with the constitutionality of certain aspects of Indiana's system for pretrial commitment of one accused of crime. Petitioner, Theon Jackson, is a mentally defective deaf mute with a mental level of a preschool child. He cannot read, write, or otherwise communicate except through limited sign language. In May 1968, at age 27, he was charged in the Criminal Court of Marion County, Indiana, with separate robberies of two women. The offenses were alleged to have occurred the preceding July. The first involved property (a purse and its contents) of the value of four dollars. The second concerned five dollars in money. The record sheds no light on these charges since, upon receipt of not-guilty pleas from Jackson, the trial court set in motion the Indiana procedures for determining his competency to stand trial.

As Indiana statute requires, the court appointed two psychiatrists to examine Jackson. A competency hearing was subsequently held at which petitioner was represented by counsel. The court received the examining doctors' joint written report and oral testimony from them and from a deaf-school interpreter through whom they had attempted to communicate with petitioner. The report concluded that Jackson's

> **Indiana cannot constitutionally commit the petitioner for an indefinite period simply on account of his incompetency to stand trial.**

---

[3] Readers are advised to quote only from the original published cases. See pages vii-viii.

almost nonexistent communication skill, together with his lack of hearing and his mental deficiency, left him unable to understand the nature of the charges against him or to participate in his defense. One doctor testified that it was extremely unlikely that petitioner could ever learn to read or write and questioned whether petitioner even had the ability to develop any proficiency in sign language. He believed that the interpreter had not been able to communicate with petitioner to any great extent and testified that petitioner's "prognosis appears rather dim." The other doctor testified that even if Jackson were not a deaf mute, he would be incompetent to stand trial, and doubted whether petitioner had sufficient intelligence ever to develop the necessary communication skills. The interpreter testified that Indiana had no facilities that could help someone as badly off as Jackson to learn minimal communication skills. On this evidence, the trial court found that Jackson "lacked comprehension sufficient to make his defense," and ordered him committed to the Indiana Department of Mental Health until such time as that Department should certify to the court that "the defendant is sane."

Petitioner's counsel then filed a motion for a new trial, contending that there was no evidence that Jackson was "insane," or that he would ever attain a status which the court might regard as "sane" in the sense of competency to stand trial. Counsel argued that Jackson's commitment under these circumstances amounted to a "life sentence" without his ever having been convicted of a crime, and that the commitment therefore deprived Jackson of his Fourteenth Amendment rights to due process and equal protection, and constituted cruel and unusual punishment under the Eighth Amendment made applicable to the States through the Fourteenth. The trial court denied the motion. On appeal the Supreme Court of Indiana affirmed, with one judge dissenting. Rehearing was denied, with two judges dissenting. We granted *certiorari*.[4] For the reasons set forth below, we conclude that, on the record before us, Indiana cannot constitutionally commit the petitioner for an indefinite period simply on account of this incompetency to stand trial on the charges filed against him. Accordingly, we reverse.

Petitioner's central contention is that the State, in seeking in effect to commit him to a mental institution indefinitely, should have been required to invoke the standards and procedures governing commitment of "feeble-minded" persons. That section provides that upon application of a "reputable citizen of the county"

---

[4]   *certiorari.* A means of gaining appellate review.

and accompanying certificate of a reputable physician that a person is "feeble-minded and is not insane or epileptic," a circuit court judge shall appoint two physicians to examine such person. After notice, a hearing is held at which the patient is entitled to be represented by counsel. If the judge determines that the individual is indeed "feeble-minded," he enters an order of commitment and directs the clerk of the court to apply for the person's admission "to the superintendent of the institution for feeble-minded persons located in the district in which said county is situated." A person committed under this section may be released "at any time," provided that "in the judgment of the superintendent, the mental and physical condition of the patient justifies it." But a statute establishing a special institution for care of such persons refers to the duty of the State to provide care for its citizens who are "feeble-minded, and are therefore unable properly to care for themselves." These provisions evidently afford the State a vehicle for commitment of persons in need of custodial care who are "not insane" and therefore do not qualify as "mentally ill" under the State's general involuntary civil commitment scheme. Scant attention was paid this general civil commitment law by the Indiana courts in the present case. An understanding of it, however, is essential to a full airing of the equal protection claims raised by petitioner.

Because the evidence established little likelihood of improvement in petitioner's condition, he argues that commitment under [Indiana statute] in his case amounted to a commitment for life. This deprived him of equal protection, he contends, because, absent the criminal charges pending against him, the State would have had to proceed under other statutes generally applicable to all other citizens: either the commitment procedures for feeble-minded persons, or those for mentally ill persons. He argues that under these other statutes

> *Condemning him to permanent institutionalization without the showing required for commitment or the opportunity for release afforded deprived petitioner of equal protection of the laws under the Fourteenth Amendment.*

(1) the decision whether to commit would have been made according to a different standard, (2) if commitment were warranted, applicable standards for release would have been more lenient, (3) if committed under [the statute], he could have been assigned to a special institution affording appropriate care, and (4) he would then have been entitled to certain privileges not now available to him.

In *Baxstrom v. Herold*, the Court held that a state prisoner civilly committed at the end of his prison sentence on the finding of a surrogate was denied equal protection when he was deprived of a jury trial that the State made generally available to all other persons civilly committed. If criminal conviction and imposition of sentence are insufficient to justify less procedural and substantive protection against indefinite commitment than that generally available to all others, the mere filing of criminal charges surely cannot suffice. Respondent argues, however, that because the record fails to establish affirmatively that Jackson will never improve, his commitment "until sane" is not really an indeterminate one. It is only temporary, pending possible change in his condition. Thus, presumably, it cannot be judged against commitments under other state statutes that are truly indeterminate. The State relies on the lack of "exactitude" with which psychiatry can predict the future course of mental illness.

Were the State's factual premise that Jackson's commitment is only temporary a valid one, this might well be a different case. But the record does not support that premise. There is nothing in the record that even points to any possibility that Jackson's present condition can be remedied at any future time.

We note also that neither the Indiana statute nor state practice makes the likelihood of the defendant's improvement a relevant factor. The State did not seek to make any such showing, and the record clearly establishes that the chances of Jackson's ever meeting the competency standards of [Indiana statute] are at best minimal, if not nonexistent. The record also rebuts any contention that the commitment could contribute to Jackson's improvement. Jackson's commitment is permanent in practical effect. We therefore must turn to the question whether, because of the pendency of the criminal charges that triggered the State's invocation of [statute], Jackson was deprived of substantial rights to which he would have been entitled under either of [Indiana's] other two state commitment statutes.

Baxstrom held that the State cannot withhold from a few the procedural protections or the substantive requirements for commitment that are available to all others. In this case commitment procedures under all three statutes appear substantially similar: notice, examination by two doctors, and a full judicial hearing at which the individual is represented by counsel and can cross-examine witnesses and introduce evidence. Under each of the three statutes, the commitment determination is made by the court alone, and appellate review is available. In contrast, however, what the State must show to commit a defendant under [the statute in question], and the circumstances under which an individual so committed may be released, are substantially different from the standards under the other two statutes. Under [that statute], the State needed to show only Jackson's inability to stand trial. We are unable to say that, on the record before us, Indiana could have civilly committed him as mentally ill or committed him as feeble-minded under [the other two statutes].

More important, an individual committed as feeble-minded is eligible for release when his condition "justifies it," and an individual civilly committed as mentally ill when the "superintendent or administrator shall discharge such person, or when cured of such illness." Thus, in either case release is appropriate when the individual no longer requires the custodial care or treatment or detention that occasioned the commitment, or when the department of mental health believes release would be in his best interests. The evidence available concerning Jackson's past employment and home care strongly suggests that under these standards he might be eligible for release at almost any time, even if he did not improve. On the other hand, by the terms of his present commitment, he will not be entitled to release at all, absent an unlikely substantial change for the better in his condition.

Baxstrom did not deal with the standard for release, but its rationale is applicable here. The harm to the individual is just as great if the State, without reasonable justification, can apply standards making his commitment a permanent one when standards generally applicable to all others afford him a substantial opportunity for early release. As we noted above, we cannot conclude

> *At the least, due process requires that the nature and duration of commitment bear some reasonable relation to the purpose for which the individual is committed.*

that pending criminal charges provide a greater justification for different treatment than conviction and sentence. Consequently, we hold that by subjecting Jackson to a more lenient commitment standard and to a more stringent standard of release than those generally applicable to all others not charged with offenses, and by thus condemning him in effect to permanent institutionalization without the showing required for commitment or the opportunity for release afforded by [statute], Indiana deprived petitioner of equal protection of the laws under the Fourteenth Amendment.

For reasons closely related to those discussed above, we also hold that Indiana's indefinite commitment of a criminal defendant solely on account of his incompetency to stand trial does not square with the Fourteenth Amendment's guarantee of due process.

Some states appear to commit indefinitely a defendant found incompetent to stand trial until he recovers competency. The practice of automatic commitment with release conditioned solely upon attainment of competence has been decried on both policy and constitutional grounds. Recommendations for changes made by commentators and study committees have included incorporation into pretrial commitment procedures of the equivalent of the federal "rule of reason," a requirement of a finding of dangerousness or of full-scale civil commitment, periodic review by court or mental health administrative personnel of the defendant's condition and progress, and provisions for ultimately dropping charges if the defendant does not improve. One source of this criticism is undoubtedly the empirical data available which tend to show that many defendants committed before trial are never tried, and that those defendants committed pursuant to ordinary civil proceedings are, on the average, released sooner than defendants automatically committed solely on account of their incapacity to stand trial. Related to these statistics are substantial doubts about whether the rationale for pretrial commitment - that care or treatment will aid the accused in attaining competency - is empirically valid given the state of most of our mental institutions. However, very few courts appear to have addressed the problem directly in the state context.

The states have traditionally exercised broad power to commit persons found to be mentally ill. The substantive limitations on the exercise of this power and the procedures for invoking it vary drastically among the states. The particular fashion in which the power is exercised - for instance, through various forms of civil commitment, defective delinquency laws, sexual psychopath laws, commitment of persons acquitted by reason of insanity - reflects different combinations of distinct bases for commitment sought to be vindicated. The bases that have been articulated include dangerousness to self, dangerousness to others, and the need for care or treatment or training. Considering the number of

> *Even if it is determined that the defendant probably soon will be able to stand trial, his continued commitment must be justified by progress toward that goal.*

persons affected, it is perhaps remarkable that the substantive constitutional limitations on this power have not been more frequently litigated. We need not address these broad questions here. It is clear that Jackson's commitment rests on proceedings that did not purport to bring into play, indeed did not even consider relevant, any of the articulated bases for exercise of Indiana's power of indefinite commitment. The state statutes contain at least two alternative methods for invoking this power. But Jackson was not afforded any "formal commitment proceedings addressed to his ability to function in society," or to society's interest in his restraint, or to the state's ability to aid him in attaining competency through custodial care or compulsory treatment, the ostensible purpose of the commitment. At the least, due process requires that the nature and duration of commitment bear some reasonable relation to the purpose for which the individual is committed. We hold, consequently, that a person charged by a State with a criminal offense who is committed solely on account of his incapacity to proceed to trial cannot be held more than the reasonable period of time necessary to determine whether there is a substantial probability that he will attain that capacity in the foreseeable future. If it is determined that this is not the case, then the State must either institute the customary civil commitment proceeding that would be required to commit indefinitely any other citizen, or release the defendant. Furthermore, even if it is determined that the defendant probably soon will be able to stand trial, his continued commitment must be justified by progress toward that goal. In light of differing state facilities and procedures and a lack of evidence in this record, we do not think it appropriate for us to attempt to prescribe arbitrary time limits. We note, however, that petitioner Jackson has now been confined for three and one-half years on a record that sufficiently establishes the lack of a substantial probability that he will ever be able to participate fully in a trial.

Reversed and remanded.

United States v. Duhon

104 F.Supp.2d. 663 (2000)

Facts

In 1997, Keith Joseph Duhon was charged with two sexual offenses after he allegedly possessed photographs of two young girls (his cousins) in sexually explicit poses. Expert witnesses asserted that Duhon was functioning within the mild range of mental retardation, and the defendant was subsequently adjudicated not competent to proceed. He was admitted to the Federal Correctional Institute (FCI) at Butner, North Carolina, for competency restoration treatment. While at FCI Butner, Duhon participated in a competency restoration group. Clinicians from that facility agreed that he had mild mental retardation, but based in part on abilities he demonstrated during the competency restoration group, the clinicians offered the opinion that he was competent to proceed.

The court expressed concerns that Duhon had simply demonstrated rote learning without adequate understanding. Two additional expert witnesses, a psychologist and a defense attorney, were appointed by the court. At the subsequent hearing, the court heard arguments about the efficacy of a competency restoration group, as well as the admissibility of testimony about a competency restoration group.

Issue

Does information about a competency restoration group meet the standards of admissibility outlined under *Daubert v. Merrell Dow Pharmaceuticals, Inc.*?

Holding

The District Court ruled that the conclusions of clinicians from FCI Butner were "unreliable insofar as it bases its conclusions on Duhon's performance in the competency restoration group." The court rejected the notion that a person could be "educated" into competency via a psychoeducational group.

Analysis

The court posited a four-pronged test for competency, based on *Dusky* and *Drope*. In addition to the well-established requirement that the competent defendant must possess both a factual and rational understanding of the proceedings, the court drew a distinction between a defendant's ability to "consult with the lawyer with a reasonable degree of rational understanding" and his or her ability to "otherwise assist in the defense." The court concluded that the report from FCI Butner failed to adequately address Duhon's abilities to consult and "otherwise assist" in his defense.

Moreover, the court reviewed the criteria for admissibility under *Daubert* and heard conflicting evidence regarding the acceptance of competency restoration groups. A psychiatrist from FCI Butner testified that such interventions are well accepted in the medical and psychological community. A psychologist appointed by the court testified he was "unaware of any peer reviews or publications dealing with the effectiveness of competency restoration groups," and he asserted such groups are controversial and "generally not accepted as effective."

The court ruled Duhon had not been restored to competency. Furthermore, given his diagnosis of mental retardation, the court concluded his "mental deficits permanently prevent him from attaining competence." As such, the court declined to order further treatment.

Edited Excerpts[1]

United States of America v. Keith Joseph Duhon

United States District Court, Western District of Louisiana, Lafayette-Opelousas Division

104 F.Supp.2d 663

June 1, 2000

Methvin, United States Magistrate Judge

Following two evidentiary hearings, the undersigned magistrate judge concluded that Keith Joseph Duhon was incompetent

---

[1] Readers are advised to quote only from the original published cases. See pages vii-viii.

to stand trial due to his mental retardation. As required by law, the court committed Duhon to the custody of the Attorney General for hospitalization "to determine whether there is a substantial probability that he will attain the capacity to permit the trial to proceed." Eight weeks later, citing Duhon's successful participation in the hospital's "Competency Restoration Group," the hospital certified Duhon as competent to stand trial. A third evidentiary hearing was held. For the reasons set forth below, the undersigned concludes that the hospital's certification of competency fails to meet the minimal standards of reliability under _Daubert_, and must therefore be rejected. The more compelling evidence, including the testimony of court-appointed experts in forensic psychology and criminal law, establishes that Duhon remains incompetent to stand trial due to mental retardation, a learning disorder, and a seizure disorder. The undersigned also concludes that no further treatment or hospitalization of Duhon is appropriate because: (1) Duhon's mental disabilities are permanent; and (2) Duhon does not pose a "substantial risk of bodily injury to another person or serious damage to property of another" within the meaning of [federal statute].

On July 24, 1997, defendant was arrested after picking up photos from his post office box, some of which depicted two young girls (Duhon's cousins) in sexually explicit poses. Duhon was subsequently charged in the instant indictment with sexual exploitation of children and receiving visual depictions of minors engaged in sexually explicit conduct.

After an initial investigation, Duhon's attorney filed a notice of intent to rely upon the defense of insanity and a motion to suppress inculpatory statements which Duhon had given to investigators, alleging that Duhon lacked the mental capacity to knowingly and voluntarily waive his Fifth Amendment right to remain silent. On the government's motion, the court ordered a psychiatric examination of Duhon. The court ap-

> **_The hospital's certification of competency fails to meet the minimal standards of reliability under_ Daubert, _and must therefore be rejected._**

pointed Dr. James Blackburn, a local psychiatrist, and requested that he conduct a mental examination and issue a report on Duhon's competence and insanity at the time of the offense. Dr. Blackburn met with Duhon and submitted two reports.

Dr. Blackburn noted that although Duhon's responses to his questions were appropriate, "many of them indicate a significant level of simplicity and/or naivete." He was oriented and cooperative in the interview, but had a "very limited fund of general information." Dr. Blackburn's report notes that Duhon initially denied taking the pictures in question, then created different versions of what happened and presented them "with a child's level of expectation that he will be believed." Dr. Blackburn's overall impression was that Duhon has "a significant intellectual deficit that precludes him from being able to totally understand the nature of the offenses against him and/or to cooperate in his defense." Dr. Blackburn suggested that additional testing be performed on Duhon beyond intelligence testing in order to measure how well he applies his intellectual ability. He recommended that Warren Lowe, PhD be appointed to conduct the testing.

In a report dated March 11, 1998, Dr. Lowe arrived at the same conclusions as Dr. Blackburn. The results of intellectual and achievement testing conducted by Dr. Lowe indicate that Duhon's current intellectual functioning is in the mild range of mental retardation and that academically, he is functioning at the age of a seven-year old. Duhon obtained a Verbal IQ score of 70, a Performance IQ of 65, and a Full Scale IQ of 67, which indicated the classification of Mild Mental Retardation. In past evaluations by the Lafayette Parish School Board, Duhon's scores were in a similar range. Dr. Lowe concluded that Duhon suffers from significantly diminished mental capacity which precludes him from being able to fully understand the nature of the charges he faces and to cooperate in his defense.

A second mental competency hearing was held on April 29, 1998. Dr. Lowe's report was filed into the record along with several other exhibits. No witnesses were called to testify. Considering the unequivocal evidence presented, the court found that Duhon was mentally incompetent to stand trial. The government then moved for Duhon's commitment to the custody of the Attorney General for hospitalization for up to four months "to determine whether there is a substantial probability that in the foreseeable future he will attain the capacity to permit the trial to proceed" pursuant to [federal statute]. The court questioned this position since the cause of Duhon's incompetency is mental retardation, which "hospitalization" presumably cannot

> *The FCI report provides no scientific or other support for the conclusion that repeating factual information to a mentally retarded criminal defendant so that he learns to retain it has any relevance to the issue of competency.*

reverse. The government was ordered to submit a brief on the issue.

On July 27, 1998, the court issued an Order of Commitment. Although it appeared both absurd and harmful to separate from his family a mentally retarded person with the understanding of a seven-year old in order to attempt to "restore competency," the court concluded it had no discretion to do otherwise.

Duhon was admitted to the Federal Correctional Institution (FCI) in Butner, North Carolina on August 14, 1998. On October 16, 1998, the Warden of FCI filed a "Certification of Restoration of Competency to Stand Trial." Attached to the certification was a Forensic Evaluation. The evaluation reviewed Duhon's background, the facts of the offense, and Duhon's course in the hospital. It noted that due to extensive intellectual and cognitive testing in the past, consistently showing that Duhon was mildly retarded, no additional tests were administered at the hospital: "Mr. Duhon's 17 years of testing indicate he likely functions at the Mild Mental Retardation range." The evaluation noted that Duhon was "calm, cooperative, and attentive during interviewing. His thought processes appeared somewhat limited but with no evidence of loosening of association or psychosis." Addressing the issue of competency, the evaluation stated as follows: "With respect to competency to stand trial, Mr. Duhon has been enrolled in our Competency Restoration Group and during that time has showed the ability to learn, retain, and relate information in spite of his limited reading ability regarding his current charges, the potential seriousness of these charges, as well as a general understanding of the adversarial nature of criminal law and an understanding of the criminal process, procedural protection of his rights, and the roles of courtroom personnel. He holds no fixed irrational beliefs about his attorney and voices a positive regard for his attorney. Based in part on our above observations, it is our opinion that Mr. Duhon is competent to stand trial."

The court thereafter scheduled a third evidentiary hearing as required by [statute]. The parties were notified of the court's intent to appoint two expert witnesses to testify at the hearing, and were invited to submit names. The court's concerns were put on record: "The [FCI] report does not identify or provide a background of

> *Courts should specifically guard against the arbitrary use of general competency assessment techniques and standards in assessing a mentally retarded defendant's competency.*

the person or persons teaching Duhon about 'his current charges, the potential seriousness of these charges, as well as a general understanding of the adversarial nature of criminal law and an understanding of the criminal process, procedural protection of his rights, and the roles of courtroom personnel.' There is no description of the information provided to Duhon which has resulted in his 'understanding of the criminal process,' nor is there a description of what Duhon actually retained. What exactly does Duhon understand? The FCI report provides no scientific or other support for the conclusion that repeating factual information to a mentally retarded criminal defendant so that he learns to retain it has any relevance to the issue of competency. In conclusion, I find that the FCI report lacks sufficient explanation and foundation for its conclusions that Duhon is competent."

After receiving submissions from the parties, the court appointed as expert witnesses a forensic psychologist, Dr. Thomas Fain, PhD, FA, ClinP, and a criminal defense attorney, Frank Dawkins, JD. It has been observed that a multidisciplinary approach is often critical in resolving competency issues, particularly where, as here, the focus is on a defendant's ability to assist counsel. In advance of the hearing, Dr. Fain and Mr. Dawkins submitted their expert reports, both concluding that Duhon was mentally incompetent to stand trial. The third evidentiary hearing was held on September 24, 1999. The government called as its sole witness Dr. Bruce R. Berger, staff [psychiatrist] at FCI who signed the certification of competency. The two court-appointed experts also testified at the hearing.

The test for competence is well-settled. In *Dusky*, the Supreme Court established a three-prong test for competency: "The test must be whether the defendant has sufficient present ability to consult with his lawyer with a reasonable degree of rational understanding - and whether he has a rational as well as factual understanding of the proceedings against him." In *Drope*, the court added a fourth prong to the test by requiring that the defendant be able "to assist in preparing his defense." Thus, to be competent, a defendant must be able to (1) consult with the lawyer with a reasonable degree of rational understanding, (2) otherwise assist in the defense, (3) have a rational understanding of the criminal proceedings, and (4) have a factual understanding of the proceedings.

Mental retardation may render an individual incompetent to stand trial. In evaluating competence, the court should take into consideration the key differences between mentally ill and mentally retarded criminal defendants. Separate techniques and measures have been developed for defendants with mental retardation. The prime reason for the division is due to significant differences between the two populations. While incompetency due to mental illness may be very different over time and may be reversible with treatment, incompetency due to mental retardation is more static and relates more directly to susceptibility to suggestion.

Courts should specifically guard against the arbitrary use of general competency assessment techniques and standards in assessing a mentally retarded defendant's competency: "The existence of a specialized competency scale for assessing persons with mental retardation does not mean that there are no other customary and accepted methods of assessment. There is a general recognition that competence is based on a specific set of cognitive abilities and the functional capacity to exercise those abilities. Thus, competency scales or structured interviews can be used with persons who have mental retardation. *However, because persons with mental retardation are cognitively impaired, not mentally ill, the strongly cognitive elements of a competency evaluation need to be given special attention. In addition, defendants with mental retardation may be limited as to their functional behavior. Thus, a defendant with mental retardation might be seemingly 'restored' to competency by instructing that individual about trial elements, but he or she may not be able to make intelligent legal decisions*"[2] [Italics in court opinion].

The forensic evaluation supporting the FCI's certification of competency notes that Duhon is mildly mentally retarded, has a reading disorder, and requires supervision, guidance, and assistance on a daily basis. However, for reasons discussed above, it concludes that Duhon is competent to stand trial. Dr. Bruce R. Berger, who signed the evaluation, testified at the evidentiary hearing as an expert in

> **The use of competency restoration groups is controversial and not generally accepted in the psychological community.**

child, adult, and forensic psychiatry. Dr. Berger testified that he interviewed Duhon approximately four to eight times and that the interviews lasted anywhere from fifteen minutes to an hour and a half. Dr. Berger also reviewed documents pertinent to Duhon's case and discussed Duhon's progress in the competency restoration group with the social worker in charge. Dr. Berger testified that at the time of Duhon's release from FCI, he believed Duhon to be competent to proceed to trial, but that depending upon Duhon's stress level and "reinforcement of learning," he might have lost capacity.

---

[2] National Benchbook on Psychiatric and Psychological Evidence and Testimony, Chapter 7 at 168 (ABA Commission on Mental and Physical Disability Law, Sept. 1998).

Dr. Berger was questioned at length concerning the competency restoration group. The report cited Duhon's behavior in the group as a key factor in concluding he was competent. Dr. Berger explained that [the social worker] developed and administered the group classes, and that he had not attended the classes himself. He is aware that [she] is an accredited social worker, but did not know whether she had a bachelor's degree. The classes take place in a 15 by 20 foot room where the group sits in a circle in chairs. Occasionally, a picture or a schematic might be drawn of a typical courtroom. Duhon attended seven or eight group sessions.

Dr. Berger testified that to the best of his knowledge, competency restoration programs are well-accepted in the medical and psychological community. However, he did not provide, and the government did not offer, any articles or peer review or other professional writing supporting the effectiveness of the practice. When questioned regarding whether [the social worker] based her protocol on any accepted study or clinical approach, Dr. Berger testified that he didn't know. He did remember having general discussions with [the social worker] and felt sure he gave her some literature. However, he stated, "to my knowledge she does not have workbooks or things of this nature. It is nearly all verbal."

Dr. Berger was familiar with testing protocols to determine whether a mentally retarded person is competent to stand trial, such as the Competence Assessment for Standing Trial for Mental Retardation (CAST-MR), and the Georgia Court Competency Test. Dr. Berger testified that the FCI does not use any such tests, and none were administered to Duhon. He was also familiar with a competency checklist based upon research at the University of Virginia which rates a patient's level of understanding from "excellent" to "none." However, this checklist was not used with Duhon.

The crux of Dr. Berger's testimony was that a person can be educated into competency to stand trial if a major problem is a lack of knowledge of the court system and criminal proceedings. While the competency restoration group also serves as an assessment tool, its key function appears to be as a forum for the presentation of specific factual information, which the patients are then asked to memorize and retain.

Dr. Berger stated that his findings were based on his individual assessment of Duhon in that he observed Duhon was "able to generate things without direct questions" and "would jump from one issue to the other so he could use some abstract reasoning that seemed fairly good." Dr. Berger based this opinion, at least in part, on Duhon's ability to discuss court proceedings in terms of an analogy to a sports game (i.e., when asked who would be the referee in a baseball game, Duhon would provide the answer "the judge"). Dr. Berger admitted that the FCI report does not address Duhon's ability to assist counsel in discussing strategies for his defense.

Considering the evidence presented, the undersigned concludes that the FCI failed to consider all four factors required by the Supreme Court in assessing Duhon's competence. As noted above, a competent defendant must be able to (1) consult with the lawyer with a reasonable degree of rational understanding, (2) otherwise assist in the defense, (3) have a rational understanding of the criminal proceedings, and (4) have a factual understanding of the proceedings. The FCI's determination of competency, as explicated by Dr. Berger's testimony, focused mainly upon the fourth factor. By educating Duhon in the competency restoration group, he learned to memorize and retain certain factual information about criminal proceedings. While there is also some evidence that Duhon perhaps has a rational understanding of the proceedings (factor 3), nothing in the FCI report addresses Duhon's ability to "consult with his lawyer with a reasonable degree of rational understanding" or "otherwise assist in the defense." A "basic ability to understand strategy" and knowledge that "his attorney was fully on his side" are not legally sufficient.

Dr. Fain testified as the court-appointed expert in clinical and forensic psychology. As directed by the court, Dr. Fain examined Duhon and performed tests to assess his competence. Dr. Fain concluded in his written report that Duhon is not mentally competent to stand trial, and testified unequivocally that Duhon was not restored to competency while incarcerated at FCI:

"It is this evaluator's considered opinion that Keith Joseph Duhon is subject to a permanent state of mental disease or defect which renders him to the state of lacking adequate ability to fully participate in his defense (both impaired understanding of proceedings and impaired ability to assist counsel in his defense). This impairment is likely a product of mental disease/defect associated with heritable/congenital cognitive retardation, epilepsy, and developed personality factors. It is this evaluator's opinion that this mental disease or defect hinders or precludes Mr. Duhon from full capacity to understand and practice daily living skills with the full culpability of a typical or normal man on the street. It is unlikely that this state of defect will be ameliorated via intervention strategies or treatment attempts. At best, intervention procedures may effect a rote repetition of conditioned verbalizations regarding the above requirements to reach competence, but these conditioned verbalizations will be hollow and without cognitive understanding or appreciation of content."

Dr. Fain provided extensive testimony regarding the specific tests he performed on Duhon and their results, including the Folstein Mini-Mental State Examination, the Hooper Visual Organizational Test, the Georgia Court Competence Test, Mississippi State Hospital Revision, and the Competence Assessment for Standing Trial for Defendants with Mental Retardation (CAST-MR). Dr. Fain's conclusion that Duhon is incompetent to stand trial was also based on and supported by the other test results, by Dr. Lowe's and Dr. Blackburn's previous evaluations, and by Duhon's school records.

Dr. Fain testified that he was unaware of any peer reviews or publications dealing with the effectiveness of competency restoration groups. In fact, he testified that there is controversy within the psychological community about the effectiveness of such programs, and that they are generally not accepted as effective.

Dr. Fain also testified on the issue of whether or not an incompetent, mentally retarded defendant could be rehabilitated and made competent to stand trial. He explained that a mentally retarded defendant with a high level of adaptive functioning could become competent. However, a defendant such as Duhon, with diminished intellect and poor adaptive functioning would most likely not be able to reach the threshold for competency.

> **The court rejects testimony that Duhon was "educated" into competency.**

The certification of competency was issued to the court pursuant to statutory procedure. Although there is little precedent on the issue, the undersigned concludes that there is nothing in the applicable statutes which exempts such certifications from the requirement that they be reliable under Rule 702 [Federal Rules of Evidence] and the standards enunciated in *Daubert* and *Kumho Tire Company v. Carmichael.* Furthermore, because the issue of competency for a criminal defendant is a critical one, with constitutional implications, it is even more important for the court to be vigilant in disallowing unreliable psychological evidence.

Daubert enunciated a four-prong test for courts to utilize in their gate-keeping responsibility to ensure the reliability of expert testimony: (1) whether a theory or technique can be or has been tested; (2) whether it has been subjected to peer review and publication; (3) the theory's known or potential rate of error and the existence and maintenance of standards and controls; and (4) the theory's general acceptance in the relevant community. The FCI's forensic evaluation report cites Duhon's behavior and responses in the competency restoration group as evidence that he is competent. However, the report contained no explanation of what information was presented to Duhon and what he actually understood as opposed to what he memorized in rote responses. Dr. Berger was unable to provide any insight because he had never attended one of the classes. Furthermore, Dr. Fain's testimony establishes that the use of competency restoration groups is controversial and not generally accepted in the psychological community.

Considering the foregoing, the undersigned concludes that the FCI report is unreliable insofar is it bases its conclusions upon Duhon's performance in the competency restoration group. To the same extent, the court rejects Dr. Berger's testimony that Duhon was "educated" into competency at the competency restoration group sessions.

Implications for Examiners

The court in *Weston* noted that the bases for Justice Kennedy's concurring opinion in *Riggins* are probably no longer valid. Clinicians can best serve courts by having current and accurate information about the potential effects and side effects of medications that may be necessary to treat a condition that makes a defendant incompetent. The courts depend on experts to explain reasons the medications are necessary and the potential effect of discontinuing medications. Clinicians should describe how medications will help because there may exist an assumption that medicine will impair, rather than improve, mental functioning. Although physicians are generally better suited to speak to the strictly biological aspects of medication, all mental health experts should be able to speak about the effects of psychiatric medications on behavior, affect, cognition, and other factors courts consider in making determinations about competency.

Even when it seems medically appropriate for an individual to be medicated, the court may not order it if other factors are not sufficiently compelling to do so. Clinicians should always identify the jurisdiction-specific criteria for the involuntary application of medicine to determine when it is justified. Generally, the courts are interested in the medical appropriateness of medicine, the probability that medicine will restore competency, the likelihood that the individual will be dangerous without medication, and the degree of prosecutorial interest in having a competent defendant. *Van Khiem* and *Weston* concern murder. *Jackson* concerns petty theft. Clinicians should be aware that the courts consider the seriousness of the crime (as in *Brandon*) in making determinations about how vigorously to pursue involuntary treatment to restore competency. *Weston* indicates that the determination of dangerousness should not be considered too restrictively. That is, clinicians should consider whether an individual would be dangerous regardless of conditions of confinement.

The decisions in *Harper* and *Riggins* provide the basis for treating, on an involuntary basis, incompetent defendants who are judged to be dangerous. In contrast, an incompetent defendant who is not dangerous presents a special case, one that the Supreme Court expects to be rare. The decision in *Sell* outlines the conditions that must be considered prior to a judicial finding that a nondangerous, incompetent defendant can be treated with psychiatric medications against his or her will. Clinicians will best serve the court when they identify defendants who will need treatment with psychiatric medication and provide the information necessary for the judge to properly address this issue.

Clinicians who are unsure whether the committing court will support a decision to involuntarily medicate should clarify immediately what the court believes the purpose of commitment to be. As *Jackson* indicates, the clinician should be closely tuned to the court's specific goals of commitment. Jurisdictions vary widely, from months to years, in prescribed periods of commitment to restore competency. Clinicians should make determinations regarding whether continued commitment will likely lead to a competent defendant. Generally, the goal of commitment is restoration of competency, not to completely heal the individual.

Duhon supports the notion that competency is more than a simple repetition of "facts" about the legal system and requires a rational appreciation of one's circumstances. Evaluators must carefully consider the scientific reliability and validity of the instruments and techniques they use to make decisions about competency. Clinicians should be able to defend their practices by more than mere claims about efficacy.

Section 5

Amnesia and Competency

Introduction to Section 5

Cases

Implications for Examiners

Introduction to Section 5

This section concerns the potential impact of the claim of amnesia on the determination of competency to proceed. The key element of the impact of amnesia on competency is how it potentially impairs an individual's "sufficient present ability to consult with counsel with a reasonable degree of rational understanding." Countering this desire to have a fair trial is the desire to provide justice to the victims of crime. Routinely holding that persons with amnesia are incompetent provides added incentive for defendants to make false claims about memory deficits. *Wilson v. United States* (1968) is a widely cited case which holds that the impact of amnesia must be decided on a case-by-case basis. The Court of Appeals for the District of Columbia Circuit considered that in most such cases, a trial could proceed if it were followed by a retrospective examination of fairness if the defendant were convicted. This decision also provided guidelines to safeguard the rights of the amnestic defendant. Likewise, in *United States v. Swanson* (1978), the Court of Appeals for the Fifth Circuit held that a case-by-case analysis of the impact of amnesia was necessary. This court suggested a broad range of questions to address the potential impact of a defendant's lack of memory on the proceedings when the amnesia is genuine. The Court of Appeals for the Tenth Circuit held in *United States v. Borum* (1972) that amnesia does not make a defendant incompetent unless prejudiced to a high degree by an inability to establish the facts of the case. More conservatively, the Court of Appeals for the Seventh Circuit in *United State v. Stevens* (1972), citing case law from the Court of Appeals for the Second Circuit, held that amnesia is not a bar to prosecution of an otherwise competent defendant.

Wilson v. United States

391 F.2d 460 (D.C. Cir. 1968)

Facts

Robert Wilson was tried and convicted of five counts of assault with a pistol and robbery. He and another man allegedly robbed a man at gunpoint, took the victim's car keys, and stole his car. The police subsequently spotted the stolen car and began to pursue it. A high-speed chase ensued, during which the stolen car crashed into a tree. As a result of the accident, Wilson suffered a severe head injury, remained unconscious for three weeks, and developed retrograde amnesia. Except for the memory loss, his mental condition was normal.

Issue

Is it a denial of due process or of the right to effective assistance of counsel to try a defendant suffering from permanent amnesia for the alleged offenses?

Holding

No. Amnesia *per se* does not constitute incompetency.

Analysis

A loss of memory should bar prosecution only when its presence would be crucial to the construction and presentation of a defense. A case-by-case determination must be made. The presence of a mental disorder is not dispositive. Nor is it enough that the evidence of a defendant's guilt is substantial. A prediction of the defendant's ability to perform the functions essential to the fairness and accuracy of a criminal proceeding must be made before trial at the competency hearing. Where the case is allowed to go to trial, the judge should determine at its conclusion whether the defendant has in fact been able to perform these functions.

Edited Excerpts[1]

Robert Wilson, Appellant, v. United States of America, Appellee

United States Court of Appeals, District of Columbia Circuit

391 F.2d 460

January 18, 1968

Before Fahy, Senior Circuit Judge, and Wright and
Leventhal, Circuit Judges

Wright, Circuit Judge

Appellant was tried and convicted in five counts of assault
with a pistol and robbery. The testimony revealed that on October 2, 1964, at about 9:00 p.m., Gerald Fells, who had just parked
his car and begun walking down the street, was robbed at gunpoint by two men who took
his car keys and stole his
car. A short time later, at
about 9:20 p.m., two men
held up a pharmacy on Connecticut Avenue and escaped with
over $400 in cash and three bottles of the drug Desputal. Soon
after the robbery a police lookout was broadcast for two [men]
driving Mr. Fells' yellow Mustang and believed to have committed
the pharmacy holdup. Two officers in a police cruiser spotted the
stolen car heading south on Connecticut Avenue and began to
pursue it. During the ensuing high-speed chase the suspects' stolen car missed a curve, ran off the road, and crashed into a tree.
One of the two men found in the demolished car was dead; the
other, the appellant here, was unconscious. Money, a gun, a bottle
of Desputal, some of Mr. Fells' effects, and a stocking mask and
hat resembling those worn by the robbers were found scattered
about the wreckage. In the accident appellant fractured his skull
and ruptured several blood vessels in his brain. He remained unconscious for three weeks. He still suffers from a partial paralysis
and a slight speech defect. He cannot now, and almost certainly
never will, remember anything that happened from the afternoon
of the robberies until he regained consciousness three weeks
later. Except for this memory loss appellant's mental condition is

> **Except for this memory loss appel-
> lant's mental condition is normal.**

---

[1] Readers are advised to quote only from the original published cases. See pages
vii-viii.

normal. He suffers from no mental disease or defect, and apparently never has.

On February 23, 1965, appellant was committed to St. Elizabeth's Hospital for a mental examination. The hospital reported that, although appellant was now of sound mental health, his amnesia rendered him incompetent to stand trial. On the basis of that report, the District Court judge held a competency hearing, found appellant incompetent to stand trial, and committed him to the hospital, where he remained for 14 months. Then, in August 1966, the hospital reexamined its position and concluded that since appellant was not now suffering from mental disease or defect, and probably was not suffering from such a disorder at the time of the crime, there were no grounds to keep him hospitalized. Accordingly Judge McGuire held a second competency hearing in September 1966. The Government's witness testified that appellant had permanent retrograde amnesia and would not be able to aid in his own

> **He cannot now, and almost certainly never will, remember anything that happened from the afternoon of the robberies.**

defense in terms of remembering any of the acts alleged in the indictment. He had "no doubt" that appellant was not feigning. However, the doctor also testified that the appellant did have a rational understanding of the charges against him, that he suffered from no mental disorder, and that, but for the amnesia and slight physical sequelae of the accident, he was in good health. On November 25, 1966, Judge McGuire filed a memorandum opinion finding appellant competent to stand trial. Judge McGuire abjured a *per se* approach to the question of incompetency by reason of amnesia, opting instead for a case-by-case determination of competency:

> "This Court holds that amnesia *per se* in a case where recollection was present during the time of the alleged offenses and where defendant has the ability to construct a knowledge of what happened from other sources and where he has the present ability to follow the course of the proceedings against him and discuss them rationally with his attorney does not constitute incompetency *per se*, and that a loss of memory should bar prosecution only when its presence would in fact be crucial to the construction and presentation of a defense and hence essential to the fairness and accuracy of the proceedings. The rule to be applied in this case is whether insufficient information concerning the events at the time of the commission of the crime and evidence relating thereto is available to the defense so that it can be said that the presence of such an amnesia as we have here

precipitates a situation in which defendant's memory is indeed a faculty crucial to the construction and presentation of his defense."

He concluded that, because "there has been no showing of the unavailability from sources extrinsic to the defendant of substantially the same information that his present independent recollections could provide if functioning, defendant's motion to be adjudged incompetent to stand trial is denied." Judge McGuire left open to defense counsel renewal of his claim of incompetence if formal discovery and other sources of information did not disclose sufficient facts to enable appellant to receive a fair trial. Appellant renewed his claim of incompetency before trial, but the trial judge found appellant competent. He was then tried without a jury and convicted.

We agree with Judge McGuire's general approach to assessing the question of competency. However, we remand to the trial judge for more extensive post-trial findings on the question of whether the appellant's loss of memory did in fact deprive him of the fair trial and effective assistance of counsel to which the Fifth and Sixth Amendments[2] entitle him. As Judge McGuire said, the question must come down to whether, "in the light of the personal intellectual or emotional deficiencies of the accused he can perform the functions essential to the fairness and accuracy of the particular proceedings in which he is presently involved."

Nor is it enough that the evidence of the defendant's guilt is substantial. He is entitled to a fair trial as well as a trial in which he is proven guilty. To have a fair trial the defendant must be competent to stand trial. A prediction of the amnesic defendant's ability to perform these functions must, of course, be made before trial at the competency hearing. But where the case is allowed to go to trial, at its conclusion the trial judge should determine whether the defendant has in fact been able to perform these functions. He should, before imposing sentence,

> **The trial judge should determine if appellant's loss of memory did in fact deprive him of the fair trial and effective assistance of counsel.**

make detailed written findings, after taking any additional evidence deemed necessary, concerning the effect of the amnesia on the fairness of the trial.

In making these findings the court should consider the following factors: (1) The extent to which the amnesia affected the de-

---

[2] Fifth and Sixth Amendments. See Appendix B (pp. 261-262).

fendant's ability to consult with and assist his lawyer. (2) The extent to which the amnesia affected the defendant's ability to testify in his own behalf. (3) The extent to which the evidence in suit could be extrinsically reconstructed in view of the defendant's amnesia. Such evidence would include evidence relating to the crime itself as well as any reasonably possible alibi. (4) The extent to which the Government assisted the defendant and his counsel in that reconstruction. (5) The strength of the prosecutor's case. Most important here will be whether the Government's case is such as to negate all reasonable hypotheses of innocence. If there is any substantial possibility that the accused could, but for his amnesia, establish an alibi or other defense, it should be presumed that he would have been able to do so. (6) Any other facts and circumstances which would indicate whether or not the defendant had a fair trial.

It would of course be desirable that defendants not only be competent to stand trial, but also have present awareness of their whereabouts and activities at the time of the crime of which they are accused. But courts have not considered such awareness as an essential ingredient of competence itself. As Judge Leventhal points out, the man accused of committing a crime while drunk may have no recollection concerning the alleged events. And in the so-called "delayed arrest" narcotics cases, while the guilty man may remember his crime, the innocent accused may remember nothing at all about his activities at the critical time. Yet this court, while acknowledging that a delayed arrest may entail loss of memory, has never considered such lack of memory as going directly to competence to stand trial.

Leventhal, Concurring

The matter must be put in terms of what is reasonable; obviously it is always possible that the defendant, if not deprived of memory, could have taken the stand and used words which, if believed, would have constituted some sort of defense. For example it is possible that the defendant might have testified that his dead companion had used physical coercion. The findings of the trial judge that he saw no "conceivable defense" is to be taken in its substantial intention - that he saw no reasonable possibility that the appellant could have given testimony that would exculpate him in the eyes of the law.

It is always possible that a defendant could gain an acquittal by perjuring himself, or more conscionably by presenting such a sympathetic figure on the witness stand that the jury would have used the mercy-dispensing power that it has in fact, though not in law. But such possibilities of prejudice, however realistic, do not suffice to prohibit the entry of a judgment on a verdict of guilty.

I don't think appellant has shown that his constitutional rights have been violated. The fact that he has no memory as to the events brought out at trial does not mean that he lacks present competency. I don't see that he is significantly different from a defendant who was so intoxicated that he "passed out on his feet" at the critical time, and does not now have the slightest recollection with which he can give his counsel as to what he was doing at that critical time. Whether a defendant's lack of memory of what he did is due to the fact that he was too drunk at the time, or ran into a tree ten minutes later, I think he can rightly be held to account - and be asked to hold himself to account if he is a man of conscience - provided the evidence is clear on what he did. It is probably commonplace for a man to be convicted of negligent homicide although in fact his memory of the event is vitiated by drink, shock, or both, and I see nothing unconscionable in this.

Fahy, Dissenting

I assume as does the court that the evidence at trial was sufficient to sustain the conviction. This is often true notwithstanding a conviction cannot stand because obtained in violation of due process of law, the right to the effective assistance of counsel, or for some other error. I think this is such a conviction. Moreover, some situations arise which place a case beyond the reach of the law we administer. I think this is also such a situation. It is unique in rarity. In the automobile crash which followed the robbery one of the two occupants of the car was killed. Appellant suffered the grave injuries described in the court's opinion. A consequence is the complete and permanent deprivation of all knowledge of anything for a period extending from two hours preceding the robbery until three weeks after it. This is conceded by the United States. Of course he would not be relieved of responsibility because of these injuries if he were in a position to be tried consistently with our system of law. In my opinion he is not in such a position.

> *It is probably commonplace for a man to be convicted of negligent homicide although in fact his memory of the event is vitiated by drink, shock, or both, and I see nothing unconscionable in this. (Leventhal, concurring)*

Appellant by reason of physical brain injury has not simply been completely and permanently deprived of all knowledge of the robbery itself but of all knowledge of anything covering the entire period surrounding it. To try him for crimes which occurred during this period is thus to try him for something about which he is mentally absent altogether, and this for a cause not attributable to his voluntary conduct. The effect is very much as though he were tried in absentia notwithstanding his physical presence at the time of trial.

We have held that memory is an essential element of competency to stand trial. While appellant's amnesia is due to physical brain injury rather than a different kind of mental disorder, this should not differentiate his case, in passing upon his ability to be fairly tried, from the case of one whose lack of memory is due to mental illness. The above bases for my view on the due process issue bring the trial also into conflict with appellant's right to the effective assistance of counsel guaranteed by the Sixth Amendment.[3] Appellant presumably is competent to observe and in one sense to understand at trial what is then taking place, but he is unable to understand its factual basis since he completely lacks all knowledge bearing on the testimony concerning his whereabouts, condition, and actions for the period of several hours preceding, during, and for weeks after the events being described at trial. Thus, he cannot provide his counsel with information which might assist counsel in defending him.

In [*United States v. Chisolm*] the court pointed out that a defendant must be able to furnish his counsel with "all the material facts bearing upon the criminal act charged against him and material to repel the incriminating evidence." Appellant is helpless to do this. He is unable to provide any facts and events of his life during the period when the crimes with which he is charged were allegedly committed. The *Chisolm* court, referring to "the language of the old books," recognized as a reason why an incompetent person is not forced to stand trial, that "there may be circumstances lying in his private knowledge which would prove him innocent of his legal irresponsibility, of which he can have no advantage, because they are not known to persons who undertake his defense."

The remand proceedings required by the court cannot solve the problem presented by this case. Appellant will no more be able to assist his counsel, and his counsel will no more be able

---

[3] Sixth Amendment. See Appendix B (pp. 261-262).

effectively to assist him, at the remand hearing than at the trial itself.

Determination of guilt is not the test of the validity of a criminal conviction under our system of law. Though such a determination is essential, it must be reached at a trial which conforms with the requirements of the Bill of Rights. Ascertainment of guilt even to a scientific or mathematical certainty does not alone suffice. The plan of the majority to have a hearing at which the Government must prove its case beyond "all reasonable hypotheses of innocence" is no more than a different standard by which to judge the issue of guilt which has already been determined at trial. It does not cure the lack of the constitutional guarantees of due process of law and the right to the effective assistance of counsel.

The rare situation before us is unlike the "drunk" and "delayed arrest" narcotics cases referred to by my brethren. A separate body of law has developed on the effect of drunkenness on responsibility for crime. For example, where specific intent is an ingredient of the offense, drunkenness is material, and so too where premeditation is an ingredient. The accused is triable for crime though the degree of his responsibility might be affected.

Memory is an essential element of competency to stand trial. (Fahy, dissenting)

He can assist counsel and counsel can assist him. I know of no case in which it has been held that drunkenness has erased all memory of the crime imputed to the person on trial, a conceded phenomenon in our case.

The present case is distinguishable in another respect from those involving drunkenness. "Amnesia cannot truly be voluntary unless it results from conduct voluntarily undertaken with the intent of destroying a memory or at least with the knowledge that amnesia will probably result" (71 Yale LJ 109, 125). It is not contended that appellant intended to destroy his memory or had any reason to believe the culmination of his conduct would be the complete and permanent loss of his ability to recall the events of a three-week period. A reasonably foreseeable result of voluntarily drinking is the lessening of ability to recall events.

United States v. Swanson

572 F.2d 523 (5th Cir., 1978)

Facts

Jack Phipps and Roger Swanson were jointly indicted and convicted of conspiracy and extortion through the mail. On appeal, Phipps' primary contention was that the trial court erred in refusing to grant a continuance because his amnesia concerning the events constituting the crime rendered him incompetent to stand trial.

Issue

What is the effect of amnesia on a defendant's competency to stand trial?

Holding

The effect of amnesia on competency should be determined according to the circumstances of each individual case. A finding of amnesia *per se* does not necessarily mandate a finding of incompetence or a granting of a continuance.

Analysis

The court specifically declined to hold that amnesia *per se* constitutes incompetency to stand trial, noting that the fundamental fairness of trying a defendant with amnesia may vary depending on the crime and the circumstances surrounding the claimed loss of memory. The court suggested no standard procedural approach in making this determination, holding instead that the standard for determining the competency of an amnestic defendant must remain flexible, as amnesia is a complex condition that may be caused by a variety of factors.

An inquiry into an amnestic defendant's competency may proceed on two levels. First, the court may apply the *Dusky* standard to the defendant's present ability to consult with counsel and understand the proceedings. Second, in evaluating whether the trial should proceed, the court may also consider other factors relevant to the defendant's particular situation. The court suggested that

these factors might include: (1) whether the defendant has sufficient present ability to testify on matters other than the amnestic
event; (2) whether the defendant suffers from some other mental
disorder that hinders present ability to participate in a defense;
(3) whether a continuance is likely to result in competency; and
(4) whether the defendant can receive a fair trial despite his or
her amnesia.

It was noted that the evaluation process will begin with a decision regarding whether to order a competency hearing. Additionally, the court noted that it may become apparent during the
course of the trial that the accused is incompetent to proceed. Because competency is an essential consideration in the fairness of a
trial, the court may at any time during or after the trial reevalu-
ate the competency of the accused, with or without a motion by
counsel.

Edited Excerpts[1]

United States of America,
Plaintiff-Appellee, v. Robert Hilton Swanson and
Jack Lavoied Phipps, Defendants-Appellants

United States Court of Appeals for the Fifth Circuit

Appeals from the United States District Court for the
Northern District of Georgia

372 F.2d 523

May 5, 1978

Before Jones, Godbold and Gee, Circuit Judges

Godbold, Circuit Judge

Phipps and Swanson were jointly indicted and convicted of
conspiracy and extortion through the mails. Swanson alleges that
the evidence was insufficient to support his conviction. We affirm
the convictions.

On February 12, 1976, 28 residents of LaGrange, Georgia,
received threatening letters, each stating that a member of the
addressee's family would meet a "FATEL accident" if the ad-

---

[1] Readers are advised to quote only from the original published cases. See pages
vii-viii.

dressee did not give $1,000 per month to "a man sent by our company." These frightening communications were the product of what appears from the record to be almost casual planning and participation.

Swanson and Phipps had been introduced by a mutual acquaintance, Adamson. On approximately January 17, 1976, Swanson received a phone call from an unnamed person whom he later identified as Phipps. The caller stated that he had a $2,000 per month job for

> **Phipps contends amnesia concerning the events constituting the crime rendered him incompetent to stand trial.**

Swanson. Swanson, after learning enough details to characterize the scheme to his friends as "blackmail," asked the caller to send him a letter outlining the particulars. After a second phone call, Swanson received an unsigned letter on January 22, 1976, describing his role in the scheme. The letter advised him to attempt to convince several named persons in Carrollton, Georgia, to act as collection agents. Acting according to the instructions in the letter, Swanson tried to telephone Hall, Pike, and Dobson. Only Dobson could be located, but he declined the offer of employment after learning a few details.

Further acting according to instructions in the letter, Swanson supplied his mysterious correspondent with the names of 25 LaGrange, Georgia, men with families. Swanson later discussed these men and their financial status over the phone with the person he identified as Phipps. Sixteen of the persons who received extortionate letters were on the list prepared by Swanson.

On February 11, 1976, the postmark date of the extortion letters, Phipps traveled from Carrollton, Georgia, to Thomaston, Georgia, to visit his parents. A letter mailed along the route would have carried the same postmark as the extortion letters. On his way to Thomaston, Phipps visited a former employer,

> **The government presented strong circumstantial evidence to connect Phipps to the crime.**

Charles Carter, at his home. The visit, though uneventful, is significant because the extortion letters advised the recipients to "Check the postmark date of this letter and a Carrollton, Ga. newspaper and you will realize the letter was mailed the night before the FATEL accident in the Charles Carter family of Carrollton, Ga." The letters were received by the addressees on February 12. Phipps stayed in Thomaston from February 11 until February 13.

The government presented strong circumstantial evidence to connect Phipps to the crime. The letter to Swanson and all the extortion letters bore one or more of Phipps' fingerprints or palm prints on the letter or envelope. The typewriter used for the letters was one to which Phipps had free access. In a spelling test administered by the FBI, Phipps misspelled the same words misspelled in the letters. Moreover, Swanson identified Phipps as his mysterious caller.

Prior to trial Phipps moved for a dismissal. Phipps claimed that he suffered amnesia and was unable to recall the telephone calls to Swanson or mailing the letters, although he had otherwise normal recall of his activities between January 20 and February 12, 1976. Phipps contended that because of his inability to recall crucial events he was unable to participate in his defense and, thus, should not be required to stand trial.

Phipps was examined by his own and government psychiatrists. The defense's expert, Dr. Hendry, classified Phipps' inability to remember as hysterical amnesia and diagnosed Phipps as suffering from a dissociated state.

> **The standard for determining the competency of an amnesiac defendant must remain flexible.**

Dr. Hendry had administered sodium amytal, a barbiturate, to Phipps. He testified that while under the influence of the drug Phipps was able to recall facts that, were he able to recount them on the stand, would either exculpate him or substantially rebut the government's case. The government psychiatrist did not directly contradict Dr. Hendry, although he testified that one suffering from the more usual sort of amnesia cannot recall anything that occurred during the amnesiac period. The court found Phipps capable of standing trial.

We decline, as have all other courts to consider the problem, to hold that amnesia *per se* constitutes incompetency to stand trial. Rather, recognizing that the fundamental fairness of trying an amnesiac defendant may vary depending on the crime and the circumstances surrounding the claimed loss of memory, we hold that the propriety

> **We decline, as have all other courts to consider the problem, to hold that amnesia per se constitutes incompetency to stand trial.**

of trying an amnesiac defendant is a question to be determined according to the circumstances of each individual case.

Although the competency determination cuts to the heart of the trial process, the standard for determining the competency of an amnesiac defendant must remain flexible. Amnesia is a complex condition that may be caused by a variety of factors. Because nonpathological amnesia may be difficult to ascertain, the district judge is in the best position to make a determination between allowing amnesia to become an unjustified haven for a defendant and, on the other hand, requiring an incompetent person to stand trial.

The inquiry may proceed on two levels. At the subjective level, the district court may apply the *Dusky* standard and look to the defendant's present ability to consult with counsel and to understand the proceedings against him. In evaluating the propriety of requiring the trial to proceed, the court may additionally consider other factors relevant to the defendant's particular situation. These might include the defendant's present ability to take the stand on matters other than the amnesiac event and whether the defendant suffers from some other pathological or psychological condition apart from the amnesia that hinders his present ability to participate in his defense. One important factor is whether a continuance is likely to do any good. Granting a continuance to a defendant whose amnesia has been diagnosed as temporary may materially increase his ability to stand trial. If the amnesiac condition is unlikely to abate, the judge may question whether the defendant will ever be in any better position to stand trial. A presently incompetent defendant may never be able to stand trial and may have to be released. (See *Jackson v. Indiana*.) On the other hand, a presently competent defendant whose amnesia seems permanent would not benefit from a continuance; moreover, because the continuance would delay the trial the recall of other witnesses would decrease, making it more difficult to give the amnesiac defendant a fair trial. Finally, the judge can evaluate the nature of the amnesia and the strength of the evidence that the condition is real and not feigned.

The necessity for a continuance should also be considered from the objective standpoint of whether the defendant can receive a fair trial despite his amnesia. Among the relevant questions bearing on fair trial and effective assistance of counsel which the judge might consider are these: Can the crime and the defendant's whereabouts be reconstructed without his testimony? The strength of the case against the defendant may make his own testimony less critical than in a weaker case. Would access to government files help the defendant prepare a defense? If information held by the prosecution could fill in gaps in the defendant's memory, the possibility of prejudice may be lessened.

Analyzing the district court's actions in the light of what we have said, we find no reversible error. We conclude that Phipps was able to consult with counsel and to participate in his defense and that he received a fair trial.

Both the psychiatrist for the defense and the psychiatrist for the government agreed that Phipps understood the charges against him and could assist his counsel in preparing and presenting the case. More-

> *We conclude that Phipps was able to consult with counsel and to participate in his defense and that he received a fair trial.*

over, because Phipps had good recall of events during the critical period except preparing and mailing the letters, he was able to testify and to present a case in his own behalf. Further, although both psychiatrists agreed that Phipps appeared to have suffered some type of amnesiac episode, it was possible to conclude from their testimony that Phipps could have been feigning memory loss and that, in any case, restoration of the lost memories would not materially aid his defense. The government psychiatrist testified that selective memory loss was uncommon and that if Phipps had been suffering hysterical dissociation, other symptoms, such as an alteration of his behavior, probably also would have been present. The defense was unable to refute this testimony.

In support of its motion the defense proffered a tape of the interview between Phipps and Dr. Hendry, his psychiatrist, conducted while Phipps was under the influence of sodium amytal administered by Dr. Hendry. The district judge listened to the tape, and the parties agree that parts of it tended to show that Phipps was able to recall that he had discussed the scheme with Swanson and Adamson as a joke or prank. Because Phipps had no conscious memory of the discussion with Swanson and Adamson or the drug-induced interview with Dr. Hendry, he claims that his amnesia denied him the ability to present the exculpatory defense of lack of intent. We reject this contention for several reasons. First, Phipps' attorney was able to cross-examine both Swanson and Adamson and to fully explore their knowledge of or participation in the scheme. Second, the reliability of the prank theory was questionable because both psychiatrists testified that sodium amytal did not guarantee the veracity of statements made under its influence. Finally, the tape of the sodium amytal interview further undercuts the force of the defense's theory because there is some indication that Dr. Hendry suggested to Phipps that the scheme might have been a joke. Thus, because Phipps' defense was not prejudiced substantially, if at all, the district judge did not err in concluding that a continuance would do little either to restore Phipps' memory or to further assist him in preparing a defense.

Gee, Circuit Judge (Specially Concurring)

While I concur in the majority's disposition of this case, I cannot agree that a criminal defendant's claim of amnesia must give rise to a case-by-case analysis of his competence to stand trial. In my view the accused's amnesia, insofar as it entails no more than a present inability to recall events at the time of the crime, is in itself insufficient to establish that a criminal defendant is incompetent.

As the majority opinion notes, mental incompetency under this statute may be found on a showing that the accused is "presently insane or otherwise so mentally incompetent as to be unable to understand the proceedings against him or properly to assist in his own defense." In its very abbreviated opinion in *Dusky*, the Supreme Court has said that the "test must be whether a criminal defendant has sufficient present ability to consult with his lawyer with a reasonable degree of rational understanding - and whether he has a rational as well as factual understanding of the proceedings against him."

> *I fear we are planting dragon's teeth, that in the future many defendants who do not plan to testify will advance this new bar to trial routinely. (Gee, concurring)*

The claim of incompetency, of course, entails considerations quite different from those of the insanity defense. The latter concerns the defendant's ability to control his acts at the time of the crime, whereas the former concerns our unwillingness to try one who is at least figuratively "absent" from the proceedings: just as we decline to try a criminal defendant who is not present to face his accusers, so do we decline to try one who cannot comprehend the nature or significance of his accuser's charges and actions. Clearly the main purpose is to assure that a criminal defendant can comprehend the proceedings against him and can rationally communicate to his attorney his own wishes and views on such strategic decisions as his defense may present. Just as clearly, this main purpose is not necessarily defeated by a criminal defendant's lack

> *We might ask whether the defendant's ability to assist in his own defense means that he must be able to relate his own version. The Dusky test in itself entails no such further purpose. (Gee, concurring)*

of recall about the events of the crime, since his amnesia entails neither present insanity nor present inability to understand the proceedings and communicate with his attorney.

We might ask whether the defendant's ability to assist in his own defense means that he must be able to relate his own version of the facts of the crime, either to his attorney or to the trier of fact or to both. The majority opinion seems to say that the *Dusky* test in itself entails no such further purpose; rather, the majority states that beyond *Dusky* the trial court is to consider other factors "additionally." These factors in addition to *Dusky* revolve chiefly about the defendant's ability to testify and about the nature and strength of the evidence against him.

In insisting that the trial court take into account these evidentiary factors - whether or not they are a part of the *Dusky* test - the majority opinion parallels some cases from sister circuits that are at least mildly sympathetic to the claim of amnesia as a ground for incompetence. Their sympathy, too, appears to derive chiefly from the view that a defendant's competence - or at least his right to a fair trial - includes some consideration of his ability to state his own remembered version of the facts of the crime, particularly where his entire defense must be constructed from that version, and cannot be reconstructed from other evidence.

I readily concede that a criminal defendant's inability to remember the events of the crime may indeed present him with significant evidentiary impediments in the construction of his defense - although the same may be said of the death of a key alibi witness.[2] But this is at most a ground for more extensive criminal

> *A case-by-case analysis of each amnesia claim is an invitation to fraud. A criminal defendant has temptation enough to fraud as it is. We ought not encourage him further. (Gee, concurring)*

discovery, or perhaps even for a continuance where it can be shown that his memory is improving and that a delay will not contribute substantially to the decay of other evidence. These, however, are matters for the proper conduct of the trial proceedings. They ought not be elevated into grounds for a finding of incompetence -

---

[2] In addition, I must express my skepticism that a defendant's entire defense can ever rest solely upon his ability to relate his version of the facts, either to his attorney or to the trier of fact. The burden is always on the government to present sufficient evidence to convince the jury of the defendant's guilt, and it is always open to the defendant to attempt to impeach the government's evidence.

a finding which, as the majority correctly notes, may mean that the defendant must be released without any trial at all.

I am especially persuaded of this view by two practical considerations. One is the extraordinary commonness of forgetfulness and, most particularly, forgetfulness of unpleasant or anxiety-provoking events. Retrograde amnesia is common and known to be so. In holding that a criminal defendant may be found incompetent to stand trial simply because he cannot recall events at the time of a crime, we may well make a substantial dent in the presumption of every defendant's competence. Second, I cannot but note the ease with which a claim of amnesia can be advanced and the difficulty of testing a particular defendant's claim where he asserts no more than his inability to recall the events at the time of the crime. I fear we are planting dragon's teeth, that in the future many defendants who do not plan to testify will advance this new bar to trial routinely.

I have no doubt that mental shocks alone may cause mental deficiencies quite as severe as these physical ailments. But requiring the presence of some causative physical manifestation might at least arguably give the court a concrete basis for believing that the asserted amnesia is genuine and that it may be of a serious nature; even in such cases the courts have by no means uniformly credited the amnesia claim. But where, as in this case, there is no accompanying malady and no concrete benchmark whatever, a case-by-case analysis of each amnesia claim is an invitation to fraud. A criminal defendant has temptation enough to fraud as it is. We ought not encourage him further.

I would hold that the bare claim of amnesia cannot form the basis for a finding of incompetency.

United States. v. Borum

464 F.2d 896 (10th Cir., 1972)

Facts

Prior to standing trial, Wilborn Lloyd Borum underwent a mental health evaluation and was adjudicated competent to proceed. He was subsequently convicted of murder in the second degree. Following his conviction, he asserted he had been deprived of due process of law because he suffered an inability to remember the events that transpired at the time of the offense.

Issue

Is a defendant's inability - as a result of amnesia - to furnish information as to acts and events at the time of the alleged offense an automatic violation of due process, rendering court proceedings invalid?

Holding

No, amnesia is not a *per se* deprivation of due process.

Analysis

The court noted that competency to stand trial has traditionally required that a defendant possess accessible memory, but the court rejected the argument that amnesia is a *per se* violation of due process. In Borum's case, the overwhelming evidence of guilt mitigated the necessity for accessible memory. Consequently, the court found no basis to conclude that Borum was deprived of any defense which would have been available to him had he been able to relate his version of events to his attorney. The court concluded that amnesia is prejudicial only when there are facts which would be before the court were it not for the amnesia.

Edited Excerpts[1]

United States of America, Plaintiff-Appellee, v. Wilburn
Lloyd Borum, Defendant-Appellant

United States Court of Appeals for the Tenth Circuit

464 F.2d 896

August 1, 1972

Before Breitenstein, Hill, and Doyle, Circuit Judges

Doyle, Circuit Judge

Defendant-Appellant was convicted of murder in the second
degree. The victim was Frances O. Borum, his wife. She had been
employed as a nurse at the Clinton Indian Hospital at Clinton,
Oklahoma. On March 9, 1970, she was found dead in the driver's
seat of her automobile on the hospital grounds, a government en-
clave. The murder had been perpetrated by some person who had
been lurking in the back of the vehicle. She had been attacked
from the rear following her entry into the car.

The sufficiency of the evidence in support of the charge is not
here questioned. Indeed the circumstantial evidence in support of
the conviction on the merits is more than adequate. The questions
on this appeal pertain to the mental condition of the accused at
the time of trial, and particularly the ability of the accused to aid
in his defense and to be cognizant of the proceedings. The special
problem in this regard is the alleged inability of the defendant to
remember the occurrences on the night of the homicide. Because
of this, his counsel argues that defendant's inability to furnish
information as to acts and happenings at the time render the proceedings invalid.

It is not necessary to detail the sordid facts. A brief sketch of
the background information will provide the basis for insight into
the insanity or amnesia issue. Defendant's wife had filed a di-
vorce action one month prior to the homicide. On March 9, 1970,
the day of the incident, defendant had tried to see her at the hospital but she would not see him. The deceased left work at about
midnight and her body was discovered the following day in the

---

[1] Readers are advised to quote only from the original published cases. See pages
vii-viii.

driver's seat of her car which was parked on a single lane, seldom used road on the hospital grounds. Tire tracks matching those of the car being driven by the defendant were found in close proximity - behind the car of deceased. Certain items of the deceased including a bloodstained handbag and bloodstained scissors had been placed in the back of the car which defendant had driven. These were later placed in large paper bags and deposited by defendant at a dump near the truck stop where he took off on the day following the murder. Defendant was at large for a year and was finally arrested in Violet, Louisiana, where he had assumed the identity of his brother. Some ten months after the homicide, defendant met an old friend and acquaintance and told him that the police had tried to pin the murder on him but that he was in New York at the time.

The trial court made a thorough inquiry before trial as to the competency of defendant to stand trial. Defendant was referred to the government hospital at Springfield, Missouri, where he remained for an extended period for observation and study. The hospital staff concluded that he was competent to stand trial and had legal capacity to commit the offense at the time. Following this the defendant was examined by a private psychiatrist and before trial a full hearing was had as to his competency to stand trial. On the basis of the evidence presented, it was held that the defendant was then competent.

There is no serious contention by the defendant that he was afflicted with a mental disorder at the trial which interfered with his ability to understand the proceedings and to cooperate with counsel. He maintains instead that he was deprived of full opportunity to defend himself because of his inability to remember the events which transpired at the time of the offense. Since he at trial had a mental block on these events, so he argues, he was unable to communicate the facts from his standpoint to his counsel and on this account was deprived of due process. We must reject this contention.

There was testimony at the competency hearing that defendant had suffered and was continuing to suffer a memory failure starting either just before the murder of his wife or just afterwards so that his memory would not function. The psychiatrist called by the defendant

> **There is no basis for believing that he is in possession of facts which would be exculpatory if only he could remember them.**

diagnosed this as hysterical amnesia. The doctor said that this could result either from guilt or from extreme shock, and that the taking on of a different identity could have been the result of an involuntary disassociative reaction. He further stated that this was probably associated with guilt while conceding the possibility that the shock of the wife's death could have produced it. In the opinion of the government's psychiatrist, the defendant did in fact have a memory of the details of the offense. He stated that it is not unusual for prisoners to make such a claim, and that it is not abnormal for prisoners to wish to forget events which are painful. On the question whether the amnesia was real or feigned, Dr. Prosser, the physician called by defendant made a real effort to penetrate the memory failure by use of sodium pentothal. This effort yielded nothing. However, both experts agreed that this drug will not necessarily provide an answer to the issue of whether the amnesia is real or feigned - a person bent on fabrication cannot be opened up invariably. The trial court did not determine whether the amnesia was real or feigned, but apparently did not consider such finding to be essential.

Traditionally the courts have been concerned with protecting an accused afflicted with a mental disorder from being tried while he lacks capacity and also with protecting him from being found guilty of an offense in a situation in which he lacked mental capacity to commit the offense. The protection of the law has also extended to an accused who has become insane after conviction. So far there has not been any appreciable tendency in our courts to recognize hysterical amnesia relating to the events surrounding the commission of the offense as a *per se* defense.

We are not here ruling out all combinations of circumstances as being incapable of rendering the trial unfair in the present context. We rule only in the light of the facts presented. Here the evidence of guilt is overwhelming. And, from an examination of the record, it does not appear that the defendant

> **Undoubtedly there are instances in which defense counsel may wish that their clients would have amnesia. We do not suggest that this is such an occasion.**

was deprived of any defense which would have been available to him had he been able to relate the happenings to his counsel.[2]

---

[2] In our case it cannot be said that counsel's inability to develop a theory of innocence was due to the amnesia of the accused. Full disclosure of the various FBI and prosecutorial investigations was made. But all demonstrable facts and inferences therefrom point inexorably to the guilt of the appellant, and there is no basis for believing that he is in possession of facts which would be exculpatory if only he could remember them.

Thus, we must reject the argument that the amnesia is a *per se* deprivation of due process.[3] Prejudice must be shown to exist - that there are, for example, facts available which could not be obtained from the file of the prosecution or from investigation by the defense. There is no suggestion as to the existence of a tenable defense which has been locked in by the amnesia.

Finally we note that counsel for defendant made full use of the evidence of amnesia in contending that the defendant was incapable of committing the offense at the time. Furthermore, full, complete, and adequate instructions were given to the jury on this subject. We fail to perceive any semblance of a deprivation.

The judgment is affirmed.

---

[3] Undoubtedly there are instances in which defense counsel may wish that their clients would have amnesia. We do not suggest that this is such an occasion.

United States v. Stevens

461 F.2d 317 (1972)

Facts

George Stevens was convicted of driving a stolen vehicle from Chicago to Milwaukee. Stevens had a lengthy history of drug abuse. He claimed his use of heroin and cocaine routinely induced intermittent periods of amnesia, and caused amnesia for the time he was alleged to have transported the stolen vehicle. A psychiatrist examined Stevens and noted the claim, but he concluded it was unlikely. A pharmacist reported that a person intoxicated by heroin and cocaine would be able to function in an essentially normal fashion, but might be unable to recall anything that occurred. No competency hearing was held. Stevens appealed his conviction to the Court of Appeals for the Seventh Circuit, stating the psychiatrist's report, which related his claim, should have been sufficient to trigger a competency hearing (*Pate v. Robinson*).

Issue

Is a claim of amnesia a sufficient basis for raising a *bona fide* doubt regarding competency to stand trial?

Holding

The trial court did not err in failing to order further mental examination or to conduct a competency hearing.

Analysis

The Second Circuit has concluded that lack of memory is an inadequate basis for finding a defendant incompetent to stand trial. Consequently, the only basis which Stevens cited for his possible incompetence would not justify a finding of incompetency. Therefore, the trial court did not err in failing to hold a competency hearing or to order further competency examination.

Edited Excerpts[1]

United States of America, Plaintiff-Appellee, v. George
Stevens, Defendant-Appellant

United States Court of Appeals for the Seventh Circuit

461 F.2d 317

March 27, 1972

Judges: Swygert, Chief Judge, and Kiley and Stevens,
Circuit Judges

Swygert, Chief Judge

Defendant George Stevens appeals from a judgment of conviction following a jury verdict of guilty of a charge that he drove a
stolen automobile from Chicago to Milwaukee knowing it was stolen. The defendant was arrested in Milwaukee on July 14, 1970
for carrying a concealed weapon. At that time he was in possession of the car which is the subject matter of the instant prosecution. He told the arresting police that the car was his and the reason he had no title to it was because he was still making purchase
payments. After being released from custody the defendant drove
the automobile to Texas where he was ultimately arrested. At the
trial it was stipulated that the car was in fact stolen in Chicago
on June 23, 1970.

Underlying defendant's challenges to his conviction is the fact
that he has been a chronic user of an indiscriminate variety of
drugs for more than
twenty years. The defend-
ant testified that the use
of such drugs deprived
him of the faculty of memory for intermittent, but
substantial portions of his
recent life, including the

> *In his plight the amnesiac differs
> very little from an accused who
> was home alone, asleep in bed, at
> the time of the crime or from a de-
> fendant whose only witnesses die
> or disappear before trial.*

period during which the crime of which he was convicted occurred. As to the question of his competency to stand trial, defendant urges that evidence of his sporadic amnesia, attributable to

---

[1] Readers are advised to quote only from the original published cases. See pages
vii-viii.

heavy drug use, is sufficient standing alone to raise a question of competency to stand trial, or, if not, is sufficient to raise that question on this record where the trial judge expressed some dissatisfaction with the report of the psychiatrist appointed by the court to report on the defendant's competency and also indicated some doubt about the defendant's competency during the trial.

The evidence before the trial court regarding the defendant's mental condition was sparse. Upon motion of the defendant's attorney, the trial court ordered a psychiatric examination of the defendant to determine his competency to stand trial. The psychiatrist reported to the court that, at the time of the examination (a month and a half before trial), the defendant understood the nature and quality of the act with which he was charged and the nature of his defense. The psychiatrist related the claim of defendant (reiterated when defendant testified at trial) that he was totally amnesic with regard to the time period critical in this prosecution. The psychiatrist stated, however, that in his view such total amnesia was not likely, though it was possible, as a result of drug or alcohol intoxication. The defendant testified in his own behalf that he had been a heavy user of drugs for much of his life and that he could remember nothing with regard to the time when the crime was committed. Finally, a licensed pharmacist testified for the defense that one who uses certain drugs, including heroin and cocaine as used by the defendant according to his own testimony, would be able to function in an essentially normal fashion while under the influence of the drugs but might later experience the inability to remember anything that occurred during the period of intoxication.

Defendant further urges that, notwithstanding a psychiatric report which did not find him incompetent to stand trial, there was sufficient evidence tending to call into question his competency. [Furthermore, he claims there was] sufficient uncertainty apparent from the trial judge's comments in that regard to establish the existence of a *bona fide* doubt as to whether [he] was competent to stand trial so as to require the trial judge to order, *sua sponte*,[2] a competency hearing. [Federal statute] provides in pertinent part that, when a reasonable doubt exists as to the competency of a defendant to stand trial and that doubt is called to the attention of the court, "the court shall cause the accused to be examined as to his mental condition by at least one qualified psychiatrist, who shall report to the court." It further provides that if the report of the psychiatrist indicates incompetency the

---

[2] *sua sponte.* On the court's own initiative.

court shall hold a hearing in that regard. Although there is no express requirement that the court order further examination or a hearing subsequent to receipt of a psychiatric report indicating competency to stand trial, it is clear that such would be required should a *bona fide* doubt subsequently arise during the trial (*Pate v. Robinson*). The question put to us by this argument of defendant, therefore, is whether the record reveals a basis for a *bona fide* doubt which arose subsequent to the psychiatric report as to whether the defendant was competent to stand trial.

We believe that the only theory by which the defendant could be found on this record to have been incompetent to stand trial would be that incompetence requires no more than the present inability to recall the events of one's life during the period of the commission of a crime with which one is charged. Moreover, we do not believe that due process requires that

> *How much worse off is a generally amnesiac defendant on trial for murder, for example, than one who remembers all but the dispositive fact: who struck the first blow?*

every defendant who claims loss of memory go free without trial. As has been cogently observed: In his plight the amnesiac differs very little from an accused who was home alone, asleep in bed, at the time of the crime or from a defendant whose only witnesses die or disappear before trial. Furthermore, courts, of necessity, must decide guilt or innocence on the basis of available facts even where those facts are known to be incomplete, and the amnesiac's loss of memory differs only in degree from that experienced by every defendant, witness, attorney, judge, and venireman.[3] How much worse off is a generally amnesiac defendant on trial for murder, for example, than one who remembers all but the dispositive fact: who struck the first blow?

If a defendant is permanently amnesiac, furthermore, there will be no time in the future when the court can secure the benefit of his version of the facts. The choice facing the court would therefore be that of proceeding to adjudicate the defendant's guilt or innocence on the basis of incomplete data or abandoning the adjudicatory process altogether.

The Second Circuit has concluded that lack of memory is an inadequate ground for holding a defendant incompetent to stand trial (*United States v. Knohl*; *United States v. Currier*; and *United States v. Sullivan*). Indeed, the facts of the competency claim of the defendant in *Sullivan* and the psychiatrists' reports regarding

---

3   venireman. One called to serve on a jury.

his competence and those in the case at bar are quite similar. In *Sullivan*, the defendant had been an alcoholic for five years including the period during which the crime with which he was charged (forging and uttering a United States' check) had been committed. He claimed that the amnesia characteristic of alcoholics which made it impossible for him to remember the facts of his experiences, whereabouts, and activities on the day of the crime rendered him incompetent to stand trial. The court there concluded: "If in fact the defendant had developed an amnesia preventing his recollection of the events of the day in question, this would not in itself be a complete defense to the charges. Such a loss of memory may call for additional trial safeguards in particular circumstances, as where delay in trial has caused the loss of other evidence, but we are unwilling to hold that [because] memory may call for additional trial safeguards in particular circumstances it is in all cases an automatic bar to prosecution for a crime amply established by competent evidence on trial."

We agree with the Second Circuit that amnesia is not a bar to prosecution of an otherwise competent defendant. Since the only theory on which defendant herein could have been held to have been incompetent to stand trial on the record would not justify a finding of incompetency, we hold that the trial court did not err in failing to order further examinations or a hearing as to defendant's competency to stand trial.

> **Amnesia is not a bar to prosecution of an otherwise competent defendant.**

Implications for Examiners

Fraudulent claims of amnesia give the courts pause in making blanket policy regarding amnesia and incompetency. Wilson was obviously not faking, but the claims of Phipps (in *Swanson*), Borum, and Stevens had the appearance of being rather convenient, and the courts obviously looked to clinicians to speak to the believability of defendants' claims. Consequently, clinicians should know how to properly examine the legitimacy of claims of amnesia. Commercially available tests can help evaluate suspicious claims of memory problems,[1] and specific techniques can be employed to directly assess claims of amnesia.[2] If claims of amnesia are believable, the clinician best serves the court by articulating exactly how competency is impacted by the memory loss and whether there is any prospect of improvement in memory with a period of treatment.

There exists great variability in how courts view the impact of amnesia. Clinicians should be aware that courts may consider factors about which mental health professionals have no expertise, such as the strength of the prosecution's case. To serve the court, clinicians should limit their findings to a clear description of deficits in the abilities relevant to competency that are adversely affected by amnesia, such as ability to provide information that might be exculpatory or ability to describe motives and intents. These factors underscore the necessity to defer to the courts the decision about whether the deficits render the defendant incompetent.

---

[1] See for example, Tombaugh, T. N. (1997). The Test of Memory Malingering (TOMM): Normative data from cognitively intact and cognitively impaired individuals. *Psychological Assessment, 9,* 260-268.

[2] See for example, Frederick, R., Carter, M., & Powel, J. (1995). Adapting Symptom Validity testing to evaluate suspicious complaints of amnesia in medicolegal evaluations. *Bulletin of the American Academy of Psychiatry and Law, 23,* 231-237.

Appendices

Appendix A

Legal Citations

Addington v. Texas, 441 U.S. 418 (1979)

Almendarez-Torres v. United States, 523 U.S. 224 (1997)

Baxstrom v. Herold, 383 U.S. 107 (1966)

Bee v. Greaves, 744 F.2d 1387 (10th Cir., 1984)

Bishop v. United States, 350 U.S. 961 (1956)

Boykin v. Alabama, 395 U.S. 238 (1969)

Brady v. United States, 397 U.S. 742 (1970)

Colorado v. Connelly, 474 U.S. 1050 (1986)

Cooper v. Oklahoma, 517 U.S. 348 (1996)

Cruzan v. Missouri Dep't of Health, 497 U.S. 261 (1990)

Daubert v. Merrell Dow Pharmaceuticals, Inc., 509 U.S. 579 (1993)

Drope v. Missouri, 420 U.S. 302 (1975)

Dusky v. United States, 271 F.2d 385 (1959)

Dusky v. United States, 362 U.S. 402 (1960)

Dusky v. United States, 295 F.2d 743 (1961)

Estelle v. Smith, 451 U.S. 454 (1981)

Faretta v. California, 422 U.S. 806 (1975)

Ford v. Wainwright, 477 U.S. 399 (1986)

Frith's Case, 22 How. St. Tr. 307

Godinez v. Moran, 509 U.S. 389 (1993)

Greenwood v. United States, 350 U.S. 366 (1956)

Illinois v. Allen, 397 U.S. 337 (1970)

In re A.C., 573 A.2d 1235, 1243 (D.C. Cir., 1990)

Jackson v. Indiana, 406 U.S. 715 (1972)

Johnson v. Zerbst, 304 U.S. 458 (1938)

Kenner v. United States, 286 F.2d 208 (8th Cir., 1960)

King v. Steel, 1 Leach 452, 168 Eng. Rep. 328 (1787)

Krupnick v. United States, 264 F.2d 213 (8th Cir., 1959)

Kumho Tire Company v. Carmichael, 526 U.S. 137 (1999)

Leland v. Oregon, 343 U.S. 790 (1952)

Lynch v. Overholser, 369 U.S. 705 (1962)

McDonald v. United States, 312 F.2d 847 (D.C. Cir., 1962)

Medina v. California, 505 U.S. 437 (1992)

Miranda v. Arizona, 384 U.S. 436 (1966)

North Carolina v. Alford, 400 U.S. 25 (1970)

Parham v. J.R., 442 U.S. 584 (1979)

Pate v. Robinson, 383 U.S. 375 (1966)

Patterson v. New York, 432 U.S. 197 (1977)

People v. McElvaine, 26 N.E. 929 (1891)

Reg. v. Berry, 1 Q.B. Div. 447

Riggins v. Nevada, 504 U.S. 127 (1992)

Rock v. Arkansas, 483 U.S. 44 (1987)

Saddler v. United States, 531 F.2d 83 (2d Cir., 1976)

Seidner v. United States, 260 F.2d 732 (D.C. Cir., 1958)

Sell v. United States, 539 U.S. ___ (U.S. Supreme Court, 2003)

Speiser v. Randall, 357 U.S. 513 (1958)

State v. Helm, 61 S.W. 915 (1901)

United States v. Abdelkoui, 19 F.3d 1178 (7th Cir., 1994)

United States v. Bordallo, 857 F.2d 519 (9th Cir., 1988)

United States v. Borum, 464 F.2d 896 (10th Cir., 1972)

United States v. Brandon, 158 F.3d 947 (6th Circuit, 1998)

United States v. Charters, 863 F.2d 302 (4th Cir., 1988) (*en banc*), cert. denied, 494 U.S. 1016 (1990)

United States v. Chisolm, 149 F. 284 (S.D. Ala. 1906)

United States v. Currier, 405 F.2d 1039 (2d Cir., 1969)

United States v. Duhon, 104 F.Supp.2d. 663 (2000)

United States v. Dunnigan, 507 U.S. 87 (1993)

United States v. Fontenot, 14 F.3d 1364 (9th Cir., 1994)

United States v. Gabriel, 125 F.3d 89 (2d Cir., 1997)

United States v. Greer, 158 F.3d 228 (1998)

United States v. Hall, 101 F.3d 1174 (7th Cir., 1996)

United States v. Harrison, 42 F.3d 427 (7th Cir., 1994)

United States v. Jackson, 390 U.S. 570 (1968)

United States v. Knohl, 379 F.2d 427 (2d Cir., 1967)

United States v. Rodolitz, 786 F.2d 77 (2d Cir., 1986)

United States v. Ruth, 65 F.3d 599 (7th Cir., 1995)

United States v. Stevens, 461 F.2d 317 (7th Cir., 1972)

United States v. Sullivan, 406 F.2d 180 (2d Cir., 1969)

United States v. Swanson, 572 F.2d 523 (5th Cir., 1978)

United States v. Taylor, 88 F.3d 938 (11th Cir., 1996)

United States v. Valdez, 16 F.3d 1324 (2d Cir., 1994)

United States v. Weston, 255 F.3d 873 (D.C. Cir., 2001)

United States v. Yusufu, 63 F.3d 505 (7th Cir., 1995)

Van Khiem v. United States, 612 A.2d 160 (1992)

Washington v. Harper, 494 U.S. 210 (1990)

Webber v. Commonwealth of Pennsylvania, 13 Atl. 427

Westbrook v. Arizona, 384 U.S. 150 (1966)

Wieter v. Settle, 193 F.Supp. 318 (W.D. Mo., 1961)

Wilson v. United States, 391 F.2d 460 (D.C. Cir., 1968)

Winston v. Lee, 470 U.S. 753 (1985)

Youngberg v. Romeo, 457 U.S. 307 (1982)

Youtsey v. United States, 97 F. 937 (6th Cir., 1899)

Appendix B

Relevant Clauses and Amendments of the United States Constitution

Amendment I.

Congress shall make no law respecting an establishment of religion, or prohibiting the free exercise thereof; or abridging the freedom of speech, or of the press, or the right of the people peaceably to assemble, and to petition the Government for a redress of grievances.

Amendment V.

No person shall be held to answer for a capital, or otherwise infamous crime, unless on a presentment or indictment of a Grand Jury, except in cases arising in the land or naval forces, or in the Militia, when in actual service in time of War or public danger; nor shall any person be subject for the same offence to be twice put in jeopardy of life or limb, nor shall be compelled in any criminal case to be a witness against himself, nor be deprived of life, liberty, or property, without due process of law; nor shall private property be taken for public use without just compensation.

Amendment VI.

In all criminal prosecutions, the accused shall enjoy the right to a speedy and public trial, by an impartial jury of the State and district wherein the crime shall have been committed; which district shall have been previously ascertained by law, and to be informed of the nature and cause of the accusation; to be confronted with the witnesses against him; to have compulsory process for obtaining witnesses in his favor, and to have the assistance of counsel for his defense.

Amendment VIII. Excessive bail shall not be required, nor excessive fines imposed, nor cruel and unusual punishments inflicted.

Amendment XIV. (*Section 1*). All persons born or naturalized in the United States and subject to the jurisdiction thereof, are citizens of the United States and of the State wherein they reside. No State shall make or enforce any law which shall abridge the privileges or immunities of citizens of the United States; nor shall any State deprive any person of life, liberty, or property, without due process of law; nor deny to any person within its jurisdiction the equal protection of the laws.